Cervical Cancer - A Global Public Health Treatise

Edited by Rajamanickam Rajkumar

Published in London, United Kingdom

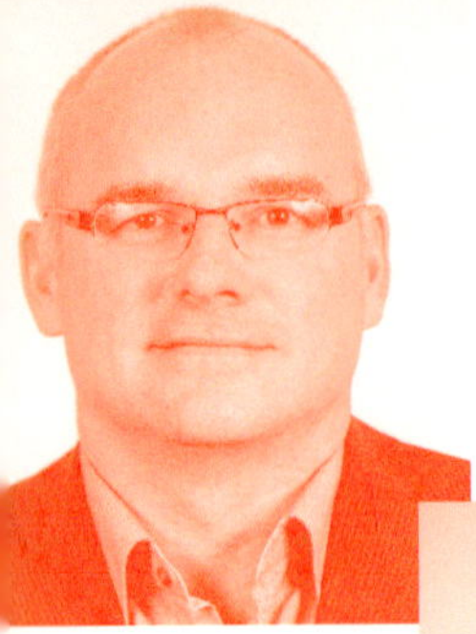
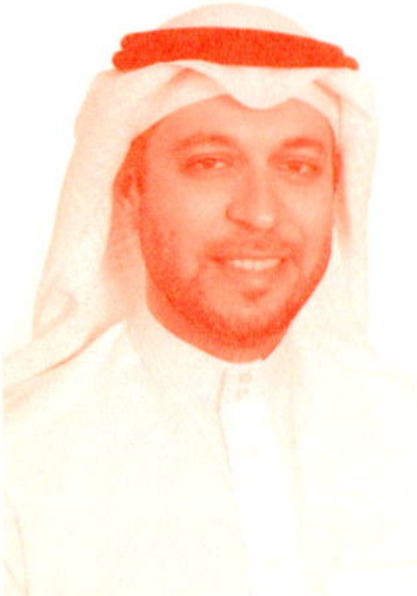
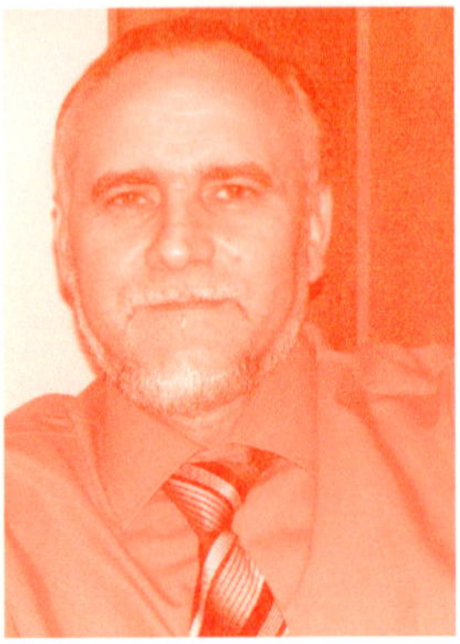
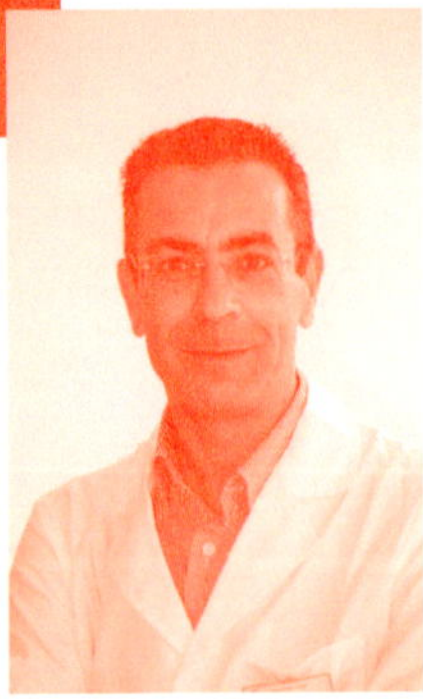
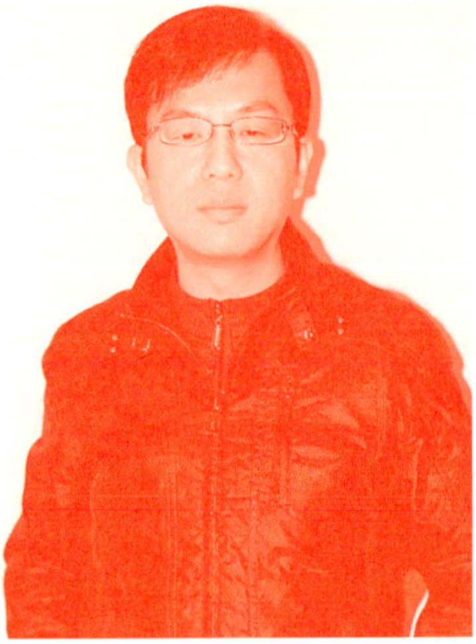
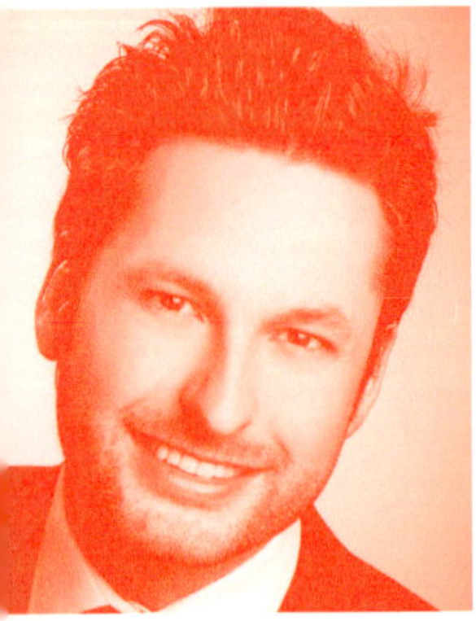
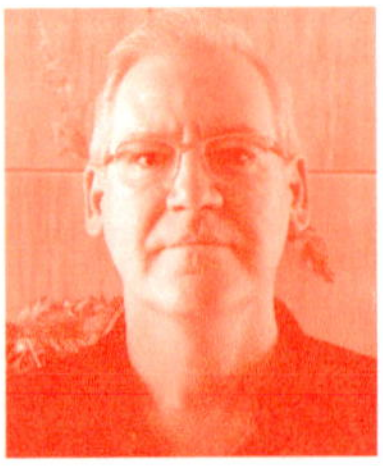

IntechOpen

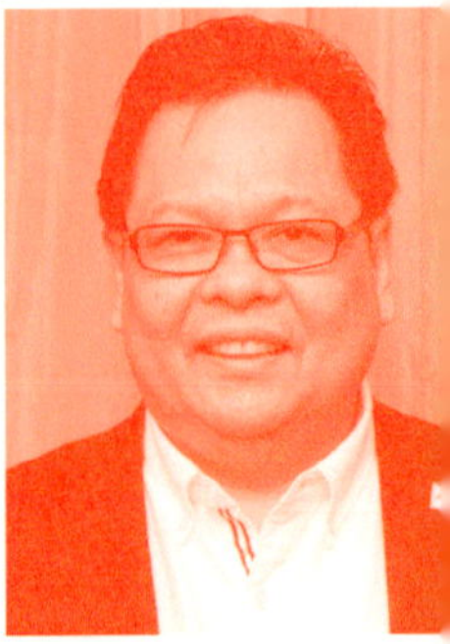
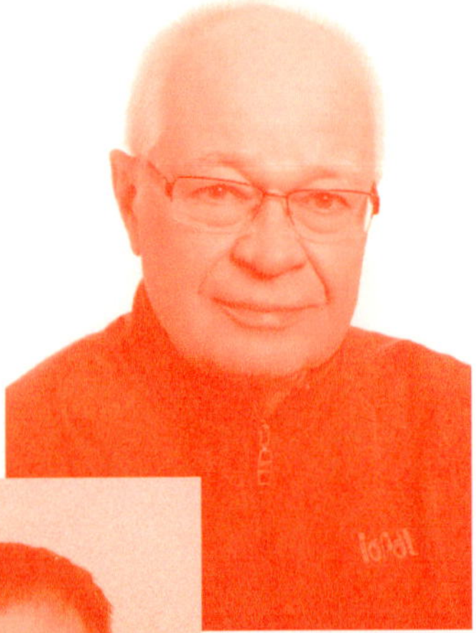
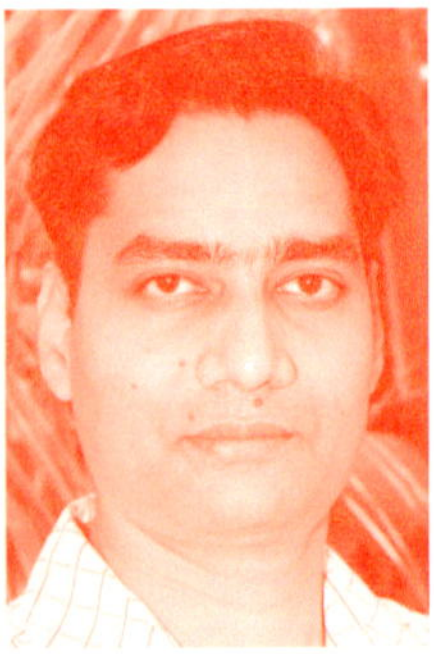
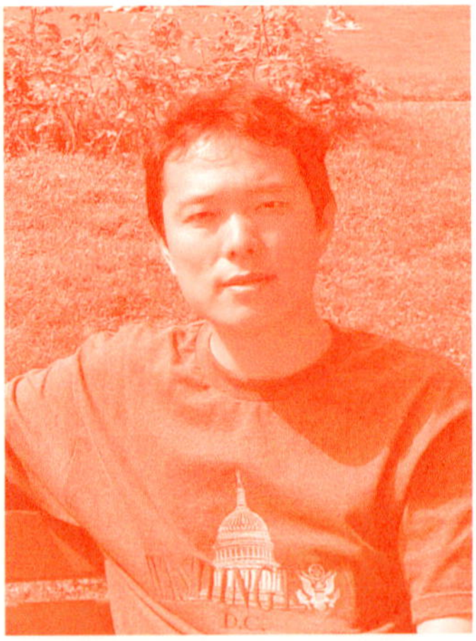
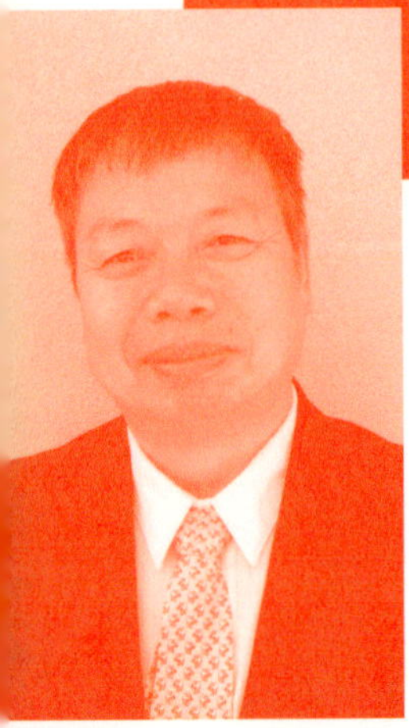
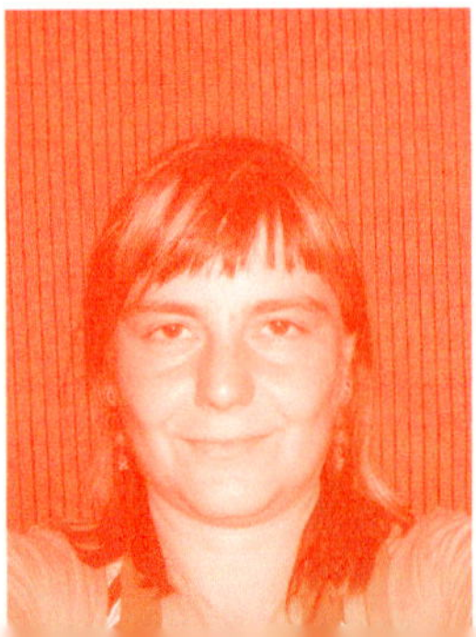

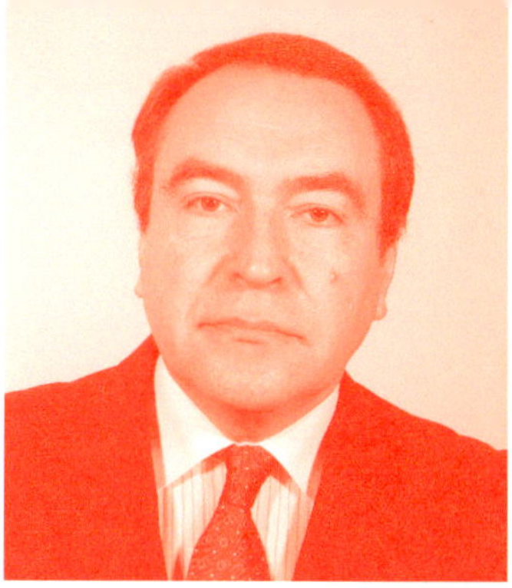
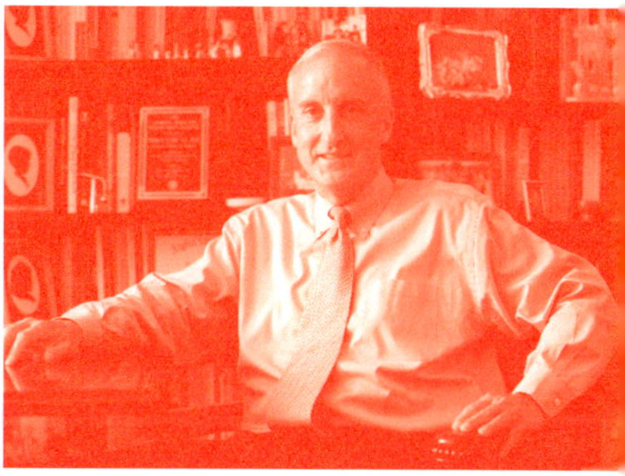
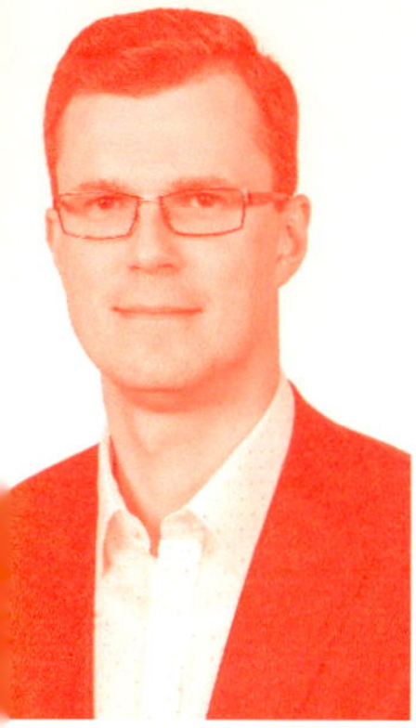
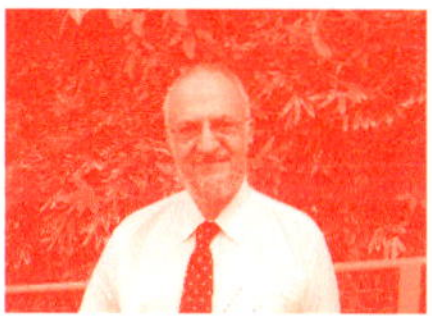
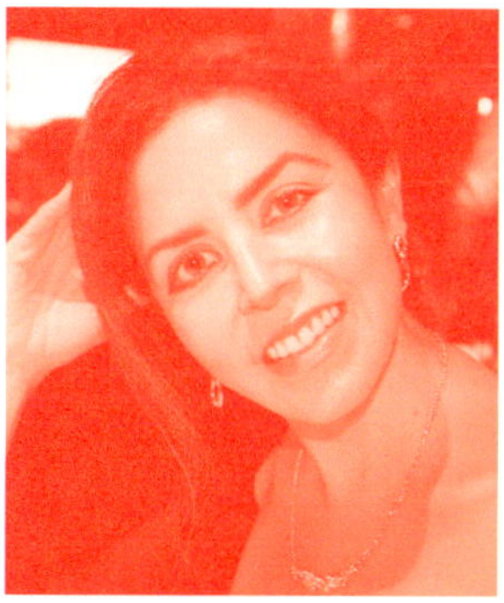

Supporting open minds since 2005

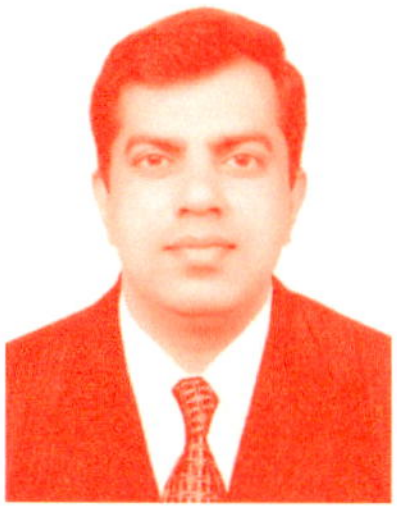
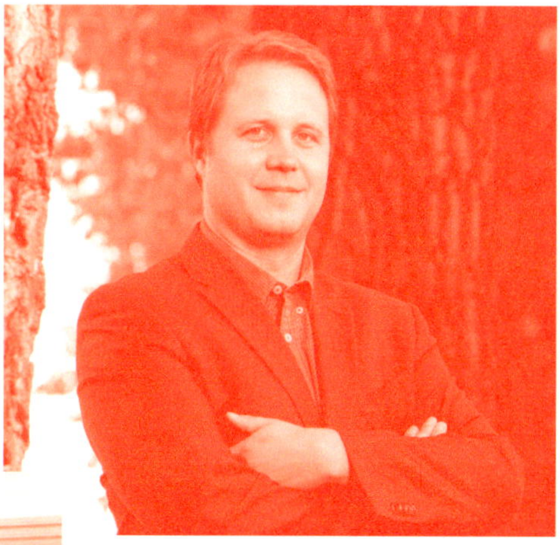
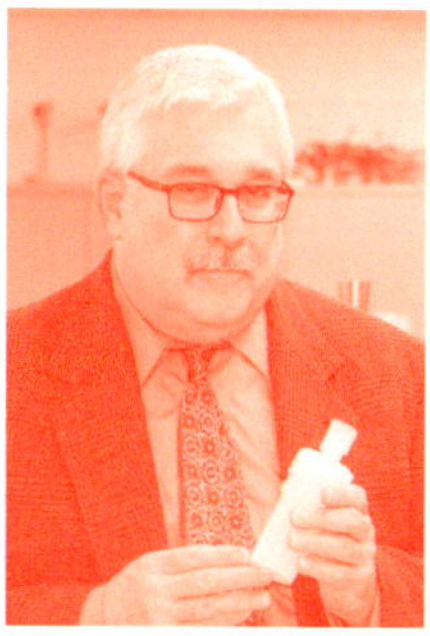
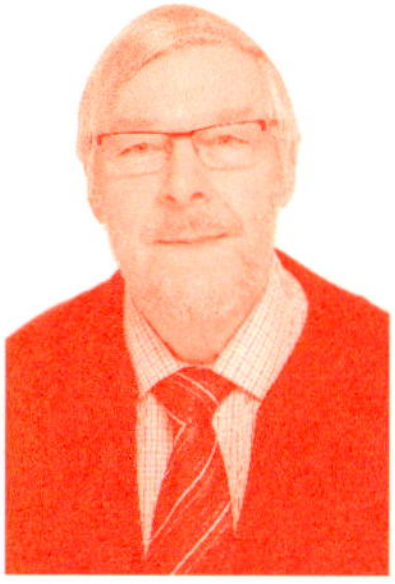
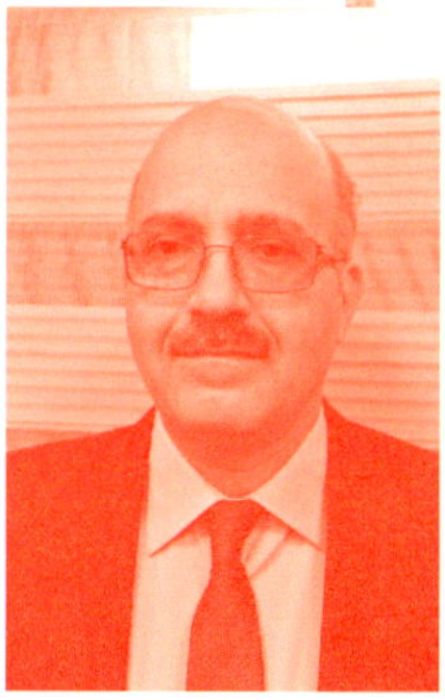
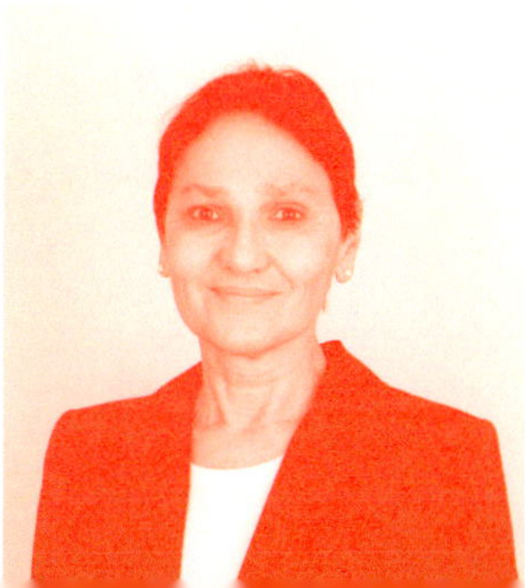
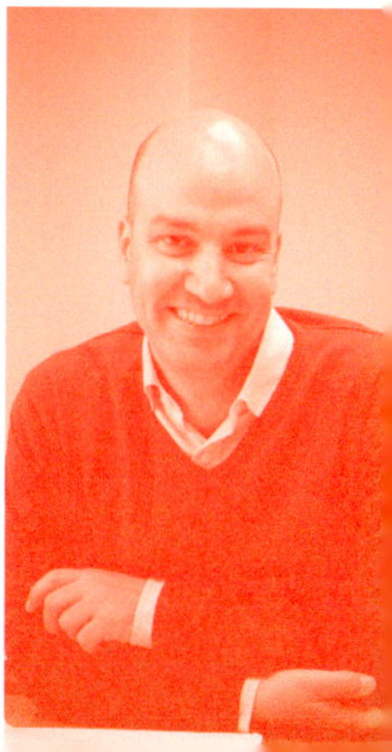

Cervical Cancer - A Global Public Health Treatise
http://dx.doi.org/10.5772/intechopen.94815
Edited by Rajamanickam Rajkumar

Contributors
Bojana Turic, Xiaorong Sun, Jian Wang, Baochun Pang, Alemnju Venceslas Tarnju, Celeste Marie Baldwin, Lisa Rinke, Sutapa Mukherjee, Elizabeth Mahapatra, Salini Das, Souvick Biswas, Archismaan Ghosh, Debomita Sengupta, Madhumita Roy, Sunardhi Widyaputra, Natallia Pranata, Ignatius Setiawan, Jamas Ari Anggraini, Maria Clara Bicho, Saliha Sağnıç, Tariku Laelago Ersado, Rajamanickam Rajkumar, Joana Sampaio, Joana Ferreira, Ana Carolina Santos, Manuel Bicho

First published in London, United Kingdom, 2021 by IntechOpen
IntechOpen is the global imprint of INTECHOPEN LIMITED, registered in England and Wales, registration number: 11086078, 5 Princes Gate Court, London, SW7 2QJ, United Kingdom
Printed in Croatia

British Library Cataloguing-in-Publication Data
A catalogue record for this book is available from the British Library

Additional hard and PDF copies can be obtained from orders@intechopen.com

Cervical Cancer - A Global Public Health Treatise
Edited by Rajamanickam Rajkumar
p. cm.
Print ISBN 978-1-78985-345-2
Online ISBN 978-1-78985-346-9
eBook (PDF) ISBN 978-1-83880-004-8

For EU product safety concerns:
IN TECH d.o.o., Prolaz Marije Krucifikse Kozulić 3, 51000 Rijeka, Croatia, info@intechopen.com or visit our website at intechopen.com.

Meet the editor

Rajamanickam Rajkumar is a scientist at the forefront of cervical cancer and HPV prevention and control. He has an MD in Community Medicine and a Ph.D. in Cancer Epidemiology. He is a professor at Meenakshi Medical College, Kanchipuram, India, and a Ph.D. mentor at Indian medical universities. He was Principal Investigator for one of the largest cervical cancer screening programs in India with the International Agency for Research on Cancer of the World Health Organization. Dr. Rajkumar is trained in cancer registry, cancer epidemiology, and colposcopy. He is also a consultant to The Ohio State University Medical Center in cervical cancer screening and an honorary member of the Society for Colposcopy & Cervical Pathology of Singapore.

Contents

Preface

Cervical cancer is the fourth most common form of cancer among women worldwide. In 2020, there were 604,000 new cases and 342,000 deaths due to cervical cancer globally. More than 70% of these occurred in the limited-resource settings of developing countries. The causative factor is persistent infections by the high-risk, oncogenic strains of human papilloma virus (HPV) types 16 and 18.

Cervical cancer is preventable and treatable. It is the only cancer targeted for elimination by 2030 by the World Health Organization (WHO). More than 193 member countries are signatories to the WHO's Cervical Cancer Elimination Initiative.

Achieving this lofty goal involves plans, programs, strategies, solutions, research, and revolutions, all of which this book, Cervical Cancer – A Global Public Health Treatise, discusses. According to the WHO, the three key pillars to eliminating cervical cancer are vaccinating 90% of girls by the age of 15 years, screening 70% of women by the age of 35 years and again by the age of 45 years, and treating 90% of women with precancer and managing 90% of women with invasive cancer.

The first chapter on epidemiology describes incidence rates and mortality rates of cervical cancer in many countries. It analyzes the sociodemographic factors responsible for the high number of cases in certain regions as well as prevalence rates of oncogenic HPV infections in different age groups and groups residing in different locations. Sex life, menstrual behavior and hygiene practices, age at which sexual activity began, number of sex partners, condom use, number of unhygienic abortions, intake of oral contraceptive pills, smoking, and family history of carcinoma of the cervix are all postulated risk factors for the high incidence of cervical cancer substantiated by case-control and cohort studies presented in this chapter.

The chapter on HPV vaccination addresses the protective value of the bivalent, quadrivalent, and nanovalent HPV vaccines and their cost-effectiveness. It also discusses problems in vaccinating teenage girls in different societies, cultures, and socioeconomic backgrounds, along with potential solutions.

The chapter on screening and treatment discusses different screening strategies, such as visual inspection methods, cytology screening, and HPV screening, and their protocols and recommendations. It also discusses treatments available for precancerous lesions, including cryotherapy, cold knife conization, loop electrosurgical excision procedure (LEEP), and laser ablation methods.

The chapter on prevention and control emphasizes HPV vaccination for all girls 9 to 14 years old and other eligible women up to 21 years old. "See and Treat" protocols, offered at least once in a woman's lifetime, help prevent cervical cancer, thus they are advocated for limited-resource settings as a cost-effective strategy.

This book reflects the rich experiences of medical professionals and scientists from various countries who are working in challenging and resource-constrained settings. We are proud to offer this resource to healthcare providers as a first step to eliminating cervical cancer worldwide.

Dr. Rajamanickam Rajkumar
Professor,
Department of Community Medicine,
Meenakshi Medical College Hospital and Research Institute,
Meenakshi Academy of Higher Education and Research – MAHER,
Kanchipuram, Tamil Nadu, India

Section 1

Epidemiology

Chapter 1

Cervical Cancer Elimination by 2030: The "SMASH" Strategy of Raj © A Global Public Health Treatise

Rajamanickam Rajkumar

Abstract

Cervical cancer is a leading cancer among women, being the second most gynecological cancers in the developing countries, accounting for about 6 million new cases every year and 3.5 million deaths. The Cervical cancer is easily detectable by simple screening tests, like visual inspection methods, pap smear examination, and the recent HPV DNA test methods. If the precancer conditions are diagnosed, treatment can be done by ablation or excisional methods. The women can be followed by periodic cervical biopsy examinations, ideally once in 6 months for 3 years. If, at the end of 3 years, there is no evidence of cervical precancer, then the women will not develop invasive cancer stages. The HPV vaccination of adult and adolescent girls, offer more than 90% protection against Cervical Cancer. Thus, Cervical cancers are early detectable, effectively treatable and successfully preventable. The author, having been the Principal Investigator for one of the largest Cervical Cancer Screening programs in India, atAmbillikai, Tamil Nadu, India, during 2000–2007, which was in collaboration with the International Agency for Research on Cancer – IARC / WHO. The program was successful in reducing the Incidence Rate of Cervical Cancer by 25% and Mortality Rate due to Cervical Cancer, by 35% in a span of 5 years. From the experiences of this "Proof of Concept" project, the author has advocated, "SMASH" strategy of Raj©, for Cervical Cancer Elimination by 2030, which is deliberated in detail, i n this chapter. Hope that, this will serve as a Global Public Health Treatise, for the health care planners and providers in particular and the community at large, worldwide.

Keywords: Cervical precancer, HPV vaccination, screening methods, Precancer treatment, Elimination strategy

1. Introduction

Cervical cancer is the fourth leading cause of cancer in women throughout the world. It is estimated that 604 000 new cases occur, every year, in the world (WHO 2020). About, 342 000 women die of Cervical cancer, per year. To stop this malady and suffering in women, and to prevent the tragic deaths, the WHO declared a strategy for Cervical Cancer Elimination CCE by 2030. There are three main targets, which will achieve that Goal.

1. To Vaccinate 90% of eligible girls against HPV

2. To Screen 70% of eligible women at least twice in their lifetime

3. To effectively treat 90% of those with a positive screening test for Cervical precancer lesions and also treatment & palliative care for invasive cancers

This chapter analysis the strategies that could be followed to achieve these targets. It is a proof of concept, "SMASH" strategy of Raj, for Cervical Cancer Elimination ©

S = Screening
M = Menstrual Health
A = Awareness
S = Sexual health
H = HPV Vaccination

The chapter explains the implementation of the above strategy, especially in low and middle income countries with limited, constrained resource settings.

Hence, this chapter and the contents of the book, serve as a "Global Public Health Treatise".

The Cervical cancer is preventable, detectable at very early stages and can be effectively treated at Precancer and Cancer stages.

Cervical Cancer is the only Cancer in the History of Mankind, to have been targeted for Elimination, at Global level.

The WHO, during May, 2018, called all the Nations, to take up the the challenge of Elimination of Cervical Cancer.

On 17th November, 2020, the WHO launched officially, the Global strategy to Accelerate the Elimination of Cervical Cancer, as a public health problem, by 2030 [1].

2. Screening

Screening is method in which, simple tests are applied to an apparently healthy women, to diagnose early changes in the Uterine cervix, the Precancer lesions, also called Dysplasias or Cervical Intraepithelial Neoplasis-CIN.

The Precancer lesions are caused by the persistent infections by Human Papilloma Virus HPV, the oncogenic strains, especially 16 and 18.

The main screening modalities are:

1. HPV DNA tests

2. Pap smear examinations

3. Visual Inspection methods by using Acetic acid-VIA, and or Lugol's iodine -VILI

There are two methods, globally followed, in screening and treatment

1. Screen and Treat approach - **ST**

2. Screen, Triage and Treat approach - **STT**

2.1 ST

Screen and treat - ST approach, involves the treatment of the Precancer lesions on the basis of the positive First Primary Test.

2.2 STT

Screen, Triage and Treat - STT approach, involves the treatment on the basis ofof a Positive Primary Test, supported by the Second Test, which also becomes positive, followed by Colposcopy / Biopsy, and, after confirmation of the diagnosis, treatment is offered.

2.3 ST

In the screening and treatment ST, approach, the women undergoes treatment in a single visit, during which, the primary test is performed and treatment is offered for the positive result. The treatment of pre cancer lesions can be done by Cryotherapy, Cold coagulation, Large Loop Excision of Transformation Zone - LLETZ or Large Loop Electro Excision Procedure - LEEP, Cold Knife Conisation - CKC and Laser Ablation.

2.4 STT

In the the Screen Triage and Treat - STT approach, if the primary test is positive, then the woman is subjected for Colposcopy examination and guided Biopsy. Depending on the Second test and Biopsy results, the woman is treated for the Cervical Pre cancer lesions.

If the Primary test is positive and the second Triage test is negative, then the women needs to be meticulously followed up.

2.5 Recommendations

The recommendation by WHO is the use of HPV DNA test as the Primary test. This is applicable for both 'See and Treat ST' and 'See, Triage and Treat STT' approaches.

In the See and Treat approach, a positive HPV DNA test would lead to Treatment.

In the See, Triage and Treatment approach, the positive HPV DNA test is followed by Triage tests like HPV Genotyping, VIA – VILI, Colposcopy, and Cytoloigy. If a Triage test is also Positive, then we proceed on to treatment.

For HPV Testing the cervical cells can be collected by the Health care workers, in clinical / community settings, with all medical facilities and precautions.

The other way is to educate women and train them in Self collecting techniques, which are acceptable, affordable and available methods.

The ideal age for screening is 30–49 years. After 50 years, if two consecutive tests are negative, screening may be stopped, but the local health policy guidelines have to be followed.

If the HPV DNA testing is used as the Primary screening method, the regular Screening interval can be 5–10 years.

For other Primary tests like Pap smear, VIA-VILI, the regular screening interval is 3 years.

Screening of eligible women, even once or twice in their life time, if effective in preventing Cervical Cancer.

Women diagnosed with CIN lesions should be treated within 6 months of diagnosis. The recommended methods of treatment are excisional, in the form of LEEP (Large loop Electro Excision Procedure) or LLETZ (Large Loop Excision of Transformation Zone). The other method of treatment is Cold Knife Conisation - CKC, and this method is preferred when the margins are reported an questionable in the Histo Pathology reports.

If there is a delay of more than 6 months, the woman has to be reassessed and treated appropriately.

Future Developments in Screening Tests.

2.6 Molecular level

Nucleic Acid Amplification Tests (NAAT):

1. High risk HPV DNA - NAAT

2. mRNA

3. DNA Methylation

4. Protein Biomarkers - HPV Antibodies, Oncoproteins

2.7 Cytology level

1. Conventional Pap Smear

2. Liquid-based Cytology - LBC

3. Dual staining to identify p16 and Ki-67

2.8 Visual inspection level

1. Visual Inspection - VIA, VILI - Naked Eye, Magnifying lens, Colposcopy, Camera

2. Automated Visual Evaluation of Digital Images – Artificial Intelligence

The recommendations of Screening Protocols have been advocated by WHO, after analysis with priority questions using PICO format (P- Population, I-Intervention, C-Comparator, O-Outcome).

The Goal of Elimination of Cervical Cancer, by 2030, fixes a target of 70% of all the eligible women, to undergo Screening, which can be achieved by using the above Procedures and Protocols [2].

3. Menstrual health

3.1 Menstrual health day: MHD, 28th may

Menstrual Health Day - MHD, was celebrated all over the World, on 28th May, 2021. This is a Global movement to create awareness on Good Menstrual Practices. This was first initiated by WASH UNITED, an NGO in Germany, during year 2014.

Every year, this MHD is celebrated with a dedicated theme. The Theme for 2021, is, "Action and Investment in Menstrual Hygiene and Health."

Removing the social taboo, creating awareness on menstrual hygiene, are the main objectives.

3.2 National period day: NPD, 10th October

The National Period Day - NPD, is another movement for Menstrual Health activities, throughout the world. This is celebrated on 10th of October, every year. The activities include provision of menstrual hygiene products and sanitary facilities. The lack of these comes under the topic for work focus, Menstrual Poverty or Period Poverty.

3.3 The national tampon day- NPT, 12th May

A women spends about 7–8 years in Menstruation and related problems, in her life time, and yet more than 70% of women, especially living in developing countries, face Period Poverty. It is estimated that more than 800 million women and girls menstruate every day. They still face the problems of taboo, social discrimination, lack of knowledge, non availability and non affordability of sanitary pads, soap and water facilities, privacy in working and educational places, and Gender Equity issues, which need to be addressed by the Government and Non Government Organizations [3, 4].

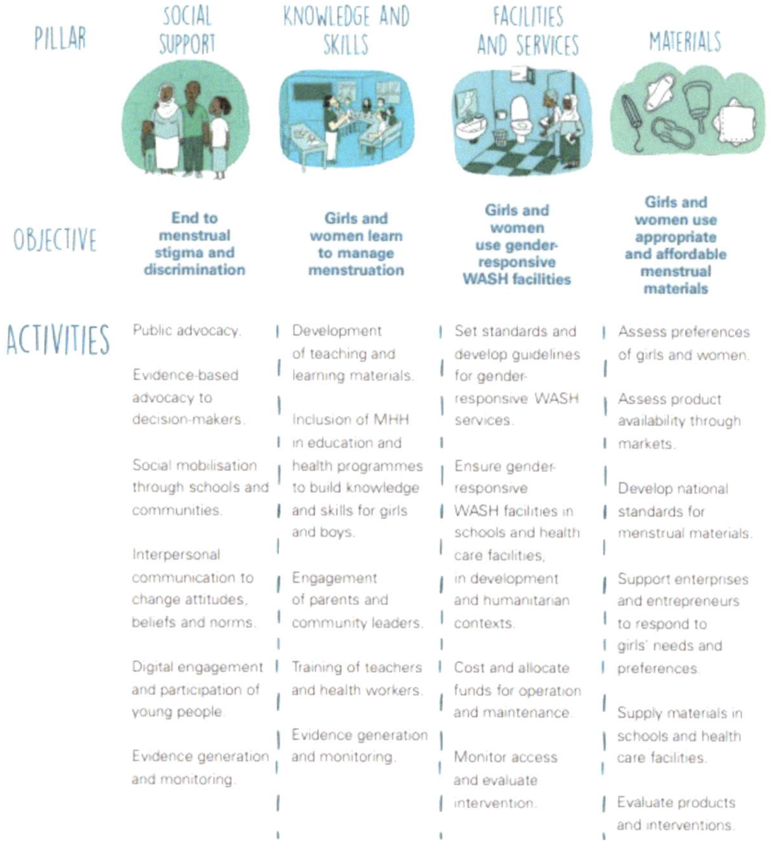

Figure 1.
UNICEF frame work for menstrual health services [5].

3.4 UNICEF: role in menstrual health

The UNICEF focuses upon the issues like Gender inequality-discrimination, Socio Cultural and Economic barriers, and to meet the unmet needs in Menstrual Health.

Menstrual poverty has many consequences like restriction of mobility and freedom in the work place and educational establishments, thus affecting their literacy life and work productivity, causing psychological problems like stress, anxiety and related disorders. To solve the problems of Menstrual Health, the UNICEF focuses on the following 4 strategic areas:

1. Gather Social support

2. Educational programs for developing Knowledge and Skills

3. Mobilize resources and develop programs

4. Provide materials and sanitary napkins and meet the Unmet needs of women during menstruation

The UNICEF primarily work through Governments and Voluntary Organizations in various countries for the improvement of Menstrual Health (**Figure 1**) [6, 7].

4. Awareness

Facts about Cervical cancer [8].

1. Cervical cancer is the cancer occurring at the mouth of the womb, the Uterus. The squmo epithelial cells undergo cancerous changes in the form of Dysplasias of various grades, in the transformation zone, which is called Precanncer lesions and later it undergoes uncontrolled multiplication called Hyperplasia, which becomes Invasive Cancer.

2. The women at risk are those who develop persistent infection by Human Papiloma Virus – HPV 16 and 18

3. The Risk factors for developing HPV infections are poor menstrual hygiene, poor sexual hygiene, early onset of sexual activity, many sexual partners, unsafe abortions, use of Oral Contraceptive Pills- OCPs, Smoking

4. Cervical cancer screening is an effective method for the diagnosis of Precancer stages. If efficient treatment is offered for the Precancer lkesions, the disease gets cured and the women never develop invasive cancer

5. Screening methods are HPV – DNA testing, Pap smear, Visual Inspection methods – VIA / VILI

6. Confirmation of the diagnosis is made by Colposcopoy and directed biopsies

7. Diagnosis of Precancer conditions are made, which are called Dysplasias or Cervical Intraepithelial Neolpasias – CIN

8. The treatment modalities for Precancer lesions are Cryotherapy, Cold coagulation, Loop Electro Excision Procedure – LEEP or Large Loop Excision of Transformation Zone - LLETZ, Cold Knife Conization – CKC, Laser Ablation

9. HPV Vaccination, for adult and adolescent girls is a sure method of Cervical cancer prevention

10. National and International efforts are made to Eliminate Cervical Cancer by the year 2030.

5. Sexual health

5.1 Important medical advice for good sexual health

1. Hygiene is keeping the body parts clean and cared so that physically healthy interactions can be made with the sex partner [9]

2. Good and clean habits are conducive for social health

3. Clean and well groomed body, helps in the prevention, cure of infections.

4. Good body boosts and maintain positive mental, psychological health

5. Good hygiene and cleanliness of sexual parts are important for safe and healthy sex, like cleaning the sexual organs with soap and water, before and after sexual activity.

6. Use of Condoms is very important and effective to prevent HPV Transmission. Also, it prevents the transmission of infections like HIV, Hepatitis, Gonorrhea, Candidiasis, Trichomonas and other sexually transmitted infections.

5.2 Oral sex

This sexual practice involves the oral stimulation of the sexual parts. Many people prefer this type of sex, because it avoids pregnancy. But due to the uncleanliness and bad hygiene of the sexual parts, many diseases are transmitted, including HIV, HPV, and other sexually transmitted fungal and bacterial diseases.

Therefore, cleaning the sexual parts before and after oral sex activity is very important to prevent disease transmission.

5.3 Menstrual hygiene

During menstrual periods, the uterus undergoes physiological changes which predisposes the cervis to invasion of organisms and infections. Therefore, its essential to maintain good hygiene and healthy practices during periods.

6. Human papilloma virus - HPV

Human Papilloma Virus infections are one of the most common infections in women in the reproductive age group. The prevalence of HPV infections is estimated to be 11.7% (Age adjusted) worldwide. There are more than 200 strains of

Type	Age of administration	Dose	Schedule*	Route	Site	Cold chain	Availability
Gardasil (quadrivalent vaccine)	Girls and women: 9 through 26 years; males: 9 through 26 years	0.5 ml of liquid suspension	0, 2 and 6 months	Intramuscular injection	Deltoid region of upper arm or high anterolateral aspect of thigh	2-8°C (shelf life: 36 months)	Single dose vial (0.5 ml) in a package of 1, 10 and 100 vials
Cervarix (bivalent vaccine)	Girls and women: 9 through 26 years	0.5 ml of liquid suspension	0, 1 and 6 months	Intramuscular injection		2-8°C (shelf life: 36 and 48 months)	Single and two dose (0.5 ml and 1.0 ml vial); package of 1, 10 and 100 vials
Gardasil 9 (9vHPV)	Girls and women: 9 through 26 years; males: 9 through 26 years	0.5 ml of liquid suspension	0, 2 and 6 months	Intramuscular injection	Deltoid region of upper arm or high anterolateral aspect of thigh	2-8°C	Single dose vial (0.5 ml); 1 and 10 vials

*Girls < 15 years (9-13 years) require two doses at least 6 months apart but within 12-15 months of first dose; girls > 15 years or immune-compromised (e.g., HIV) women require three doses for full protection. HPV: Human papillomavirus

Figure 2.
HPV vaccine schedule and other details: [10].

HPV, but the Oncogenic strains are HPV 16 and 18. More than 80% of the women have the risk of getting HPV infections in their life time. But most of the infections undergo spontaneous regression. In 1980, Zur Hausen, described the causal relationship of HPV infections and development of Cervical cancer. HPV infections cause other cancers of Oropharynxl, Anus, Vagina, Vulva and Penis.

6.1 Prevention and control strategies

1. HPV Vaccination

2. Screening

3. Treatment of Precancer lesions

4. Follow up for 3 years with 6 monthly Cervical biopsies

5. Declare cure at the end of 3 years if the Histo Pathology reports of the cervical biopsies indicate 'No Evidence of Disease'.

6.2 HPV vaccines

1. Quadrivalent vaccine: HPV types 6,11,16 and 18

2. Nine valent vaccine: HPV types 6,11,16,18,31,33,45,52,58

Protection rate = 70–90%.

The Nine valent vaccine offers protection against Cervical cancer and also, Anal, Vaginal, Vulval, Penile and Oropharyngeal cancers (**Figure 2**).

7. Conclusion

As conclusion, the author chooses to high light the newly developed, motivational slogan **"ILLUMINATE – PARTICIPATE- ELIMINATE".**

We have to *ILLUMINATE* our knowledge and skills about the facts of Cervical cancer, especially understand that *Primordial prevention,* can be achieved by preventing HPV in the community through HPV Vaccination. *Primary prevention* can be achieved by Health Promotion and Specific protection, by maintaining good Menstrual and Sexual Health. *Secondary prevention* can be achieved by "Early diagnosis and Treatment", by screening and treatment of Precancer stages and cure of the lesions, thus preventing them from developing in to invasive cancer stages.

Tertiary prevention is by Palliative care and disability limitation and rehabilitation.

The next step is to **PARTICIPATE** in awareness and health education programs, HPV Vaccination camps, Screening and treatment programs, ensuring and encouraging compliance by the community for the medical guidance and follow up schedules.

To **ELIMINATE**, is to reduce the prevelance of Cervical cancer to less than 4/100,000, by self motivation, community commitment and Global policy and political will.

To conclude, we will Illuminate, all our buildings by **TEAL LIGHT on November 17th, every year, to symbolize ourselves as Community Captains, for Elimination of Cervical Cancer, all over the world, by 2030.**

Author details

Rajamanickam Rajkumar
Community Medicine, Meenakshi Medical College Hospital and Research Institute, Meenakshi Academy of Higher Education Research—MAHER, Kanchipuram, Tamil Nadu, India

*Address all correspondence to: rajcfchc@gmail.com

References

[1] https://www.thelancet.com/journals/langlo/article/PIIS2214-109X(20)30522-2/fulltext?rss=yes

[2] WHO guideline for screening and treatment of cervical pre-cancer lesions for cervical cancer prevention, second edition, 2021.

[3] National Tampon Day - National Day Archives https://www.nationaldayarchives.com › day › national-ta

[4] Menstrual Hygiene Management Day resource collection on Globalwaters.org.

[5] Guidance on Menstrual Health and Hygiene, Unicef, 2019.

[6] Guidance on Menstrual Health and Hygiene – UNICEF – ReferDocument.

[7] https://www.unicef.org/wash/schools/files/Advancing_WASH_in_Schools_Monitoring(1).pdf

[8] CAPED https://www.capedindia.org/faq/

[9] https://www.evaidya.com/Health-Articles/top-sexual-hygiene-habits-you-must-follow-in- your-daily-life/

[10] Sachdeva S, Sachdeva R. Human papillomavirus vaccination: Review and roll out plan in Delhi. CHRISMED J Health Res [serial online] 2016 [cited 2021 Jul 24];3:252-7. Available from: https://www.cjhr.org/text.asp?2016/3/4/252/190584

Chapter 2

Global Burden of Cervical Cancer

Alemnju Venceslas Tarnju

Abstract

Human papillomavirus (HPV) has caused infections and malignancies worldwide among which is cervical cancer. In 2004 WHO reported that cervical cancer was the most common cause of cancer deaths among women in developing countries. Globally, 570,000 cases per year in women are attributed to HPV, which is about 8.6% of all occurring cancers. Female mortality is estimated at 250,000 with 80% of incidence and mortality rates occurring in Latin America and Sub Saharan Africa (SSA). Cervical cancer demographic variation in 3rd world countries can be attributed to inadequate health care systems and screening process. As one of the most preventable cancers, early screening and vaccination have shown to limit the late stage of the disease. With present studies estimating worldwide incidence at 4.5% a year. The need for preventive measures to halt the progression of a global public health concern like cancer deaths in women cannot be overemphasized.

Keywords: HPV, Incidence, Mortality, Sub Saharan Africa, worldwide estimate, Global trends

1. Introduction

Cervical cancer is the most common cause of cancer deaths among women in developing countries [1]. Human papillomavirus (HPV) has caused severe infections globally including cervical cancer. HPV is responsible for malignancy and mortality in women across the world [2] and has claimed the lives of thousands of women. HPV infections have been estimated to reach 500,000 a year, with an estimated 80 percent being recorded in third world countries. Female mortality is recorded at 250,000 [2].

Research has shown that human papillomavirus causes cervical cancer in women. Early screening and treatment reduce this cancer rate significantly, preventing the formation of late-stage cancer.

The cervical cancer demographic includes mostly women who are of childbearing age. HPV predisposition is seen in the early onset of sexual intercourse, multiple sexual partners, HPV genome, women on oral contraceptive pills, immune-deficient individuals, or smoking lifestyle. Lack of adequate health care systems leading to inadequate screening has precipitated an increase in advanced cancer that is no longer controllable and difficult to treat. Half of the female population who are sexually active and are not immunized will come down with HPV during their adult lives [3].

HPV16 and 18 (high risk strains) have been found in almost all cases of cervical cancer. Women with HPV have no signs even after infection, so early detection without screening is difficult, and so is the cancer progression. The time lag from the time of infection to the actual HPV disease or cervical cancer development takes a long time, approximately 10 to 20 years.

According to CDC guidelines, HPV vaccines should be administered to girls between 11 and 12 years old [4]. Although cervical cancer is one of the most preventable cancers, present studies estimate worldwide incidence at 4.5% [5] hence the need for preventive measures.

2. Global burden of the disease (incidence and mortality rates)

In 2012 cervical cancer was the fourth most commonly diagnosed cancer in women, with about 527,600 new cases worldwide and 265,700 estimated deaths which was about 7.5% of all cancer deaths in females. More than half were diagnosed in Central, South America and sub-Saharan Africa and with lowest rates in the Middle East, Northern America, Australia and New Zealand, China, and parts of Western Europe [6]. Present study estimates the worldwide incidence at 4.5% a year [5]. Cervical cancer is the second most commonly diagnosed cancer after breast cancer and the third leading cause of cancer death after breast and lung cancers with about 90% of cervical deaths in the world occurring in developing countries, with India alone accounting for about 25% of the total case [7].

The regions with the highest burden of cervical cancer are those not able to provide vaccines and essential screening methods due to inadequate health care system. About 570 000 women developed cervical cancer in 2018 and of that an estimated 311, 000 died from cervical cancer [8] with China and India contributing a large portion of the global burden.

3. Discussion

The Human papillomavirus belongs to the Papilloma viridae family; double-stranded circular DNA virus, protected by an icosahedral protein capsid which is none enveloped. Because there is no host genome integration of viral DNA, HPV types 6, 11,42, and 44 cause infection of lesser severity. Malignant HPV occurs when the P53 suppressor gene and retinoblastoma gene are inactivated due to the presence of oncoproteins E6 and E7. Several types (40, classified in the Alpha papillomavirus genus) are seen to infect mucosal tissue in the anogenital area and each has connections with cancer. Low grade cervical intra epithelial lesions (LSIL), condylomas, and respiratory papilloma are seen in low-grade HPV. The high-risk types can cause squamous and granular high-grade intra epithelial lesions and oropharyngeal cancer. The immune response is responsible for removing most of the HPV from the system. Types HPV16 and HPV18 have vaccines currently in use worldwide. HPV16 and 18 have cancerous lesions of the cervix in about 70% of all cases.

Women with HPV have no signs even after infection, so early detection without screening is difficult, and so is the cancer progression. It is crucial to find out the genomic types as the information can lead to knowledge of the spread, location and geographic areas of HPV infection. Different subsets of HPV16 and HPV18 have their specific geographic locations and specific ethnic groups that they predominate, whereas, in other types such as HPV 58, these parameters are not so exact. The time lag from the time of infection to the actual HPV disease or cervical cancer development takes a long time, approximately 10 to 20 years. It starts with transforming normal cells into precancerous cells and then into metastatic cancer cells (dysplasia). This formation of koilocytosis in squamous cells also called a clear halo, is displayed by the cell containing a wrinkled, pyknotic nucleus. It is however, to determine the relationship between HPV and precancerous cervical lesions.

The area of metaplastic tissue between the squamous epithelium of the vagina and the glandular tissue of the cervix (susceptible to carcinogenesis) is the cervical transformation zone (CTZ). Cervical cancer is virtually impossible in the absence of sexually transmitted HPV infection [9] and the lack of intermediate progression to pre cancer [10]. HPV infection is the leading cause of cervical intra epithelial neoplasia [11]. Patients with persistent oncogenic HPV infection usually show cervical lesion progression from low to high grade and people with higher genomic copies [12, 13].

4. Conclusion

Cancer is the second leading cause of death in women, as reported by the Centers for disease control (CDC) and prevention in the United States of America. The need for preventive measures to stem cancer deaths in women cannot be overemphasized. Human papillomavirus causes cervical cancers in women, as seen in studies of many reviewed articles. HPV cancers are estimated to be about 100 types of HPV, with many of them being transmitted sexually. HPV is the most common among sexually transmitted diseases. The most carcinogenic forms are HPV types 16, 18, 31, and 35, among others. Other HPV types can cause cervical cancers and might be responsible for a sizeable portion of the cancers. The HPV 16 is the primary type indicated in 20% of HPV infections but which causes 40% of the high grade squamous intra epithelial lesion. HPV 18 is a close second and is implicated in the formation of adenocarcinomas [10].

According to CDC guidelines [4], HPV vaccines should be administered to girls between 11 and 12 years old. Three doses of the vaccine given within three months showed a high efficacy of preventing HPV disease when they become sexually active in later life. HPV is seen when there is an early onset of sexual intercourse and when individuals have multiple sexual partners. HPV screening should be instituted at 21 years of age with a Papanicolaou test (Pap smear test to check for cancer and pre cancers in women) every three years. Women over the age of 30 should be screened every five years, and women over 65 who are negative of previous screening should not necessarily be screened. Early screening has shown early detection and treatment of HPV and thereby reducing mortality in women. The justification for early screening is to offer low-cost accessible means of determining who in the population is likely to develop the disease and provide diagnostic testing and appropriate treatment.

The recommendation is to emphasize early detection of cancer or pre-cancerous cells, especially in vulnerable or very hard and remote communities. Studies showed that half of the women tested in remote locations are unaware of sexually transmitted infections or HPV. Some of those communities also have no HPV vaccine immunization programs [2]. There is a need to train health care workers to teach communities about sexually transmitted diseases. The importance of determining genomic copies and co-infections in HPV 16 and 18 is a better approach to predict the prognosis of HPV instead of relying solely on genotyping [12]. Women with more than one genotype infections were seen to have more cervical lesions. Public health aims to eradicate HPV cancers through effective screening detection programs and vaccinations across the population. Research should go beyond initial screening for HPV and include HPV genotyping to better manage precancerous treatment plans [14]. HPV eradication should be of primary focus.

Declaration

The author has no conflict of interest to declare.

Author details

Alemnju Venceslas Tarnju[1,2]

1 Bachelors Medical Lab Science (B.MLS), Faculty of Health Science, Buea, Cameroon

2 All Saints University School of Medicine, Roseau, Dominica

*Address all correspondence to: alemnjuvenceslas231@gmail.com

References

[1] Ferlay J, Soerjomataram I, Dikshit R, Eser S, Mathers C, Rebelo M, et al. Cancer incidence and mortality worldwide: Sources, methods and major patterns in GLOBOCAN 2012. Int J Cancer. 2015;136(5):E359–E386.

[2] Fuenmayor A, Fernández C, Pérez V, Coronado J, Ávila M, Fernandes A, et al. Detection of precancerous lesions in the cervix and HPV infection in women in the region of Maniapure, Bolivar State. Ecancermedicalscience. 2018;12:1-11.

[3] Gatumo M, Gacheri S, Sayed AR, Scheibe A. Women's knowledge and attitudes related to cervical cancer and cervical cancer screening in Isiolo and Tharaka Nithi counties, Kenya: A cross-sectional study. BMC Cancer. 2018;18(1):1-9.

[4] Centers for Disease Control and Prevention (CDC). Measles - United States, 2011. MMWR Morb Mortal Wkly Rep [Internet]. 2012;61(15):253-7. Available from: http://www.ncbi.nlm.nih.gov/pubmed/22513526

[5] de Martel C, Plummer M, Vignat J, Franceschi S. Worldwide burden of cancer attributable to HPV by site, country and HPV type. Int J Cancer. 2017;141(4):664-670.

[6] Cecilia, N.C. et al. Global Burden of Cervical Cancer: a Literature Review. Int J Public Heal Clin Sci [Internet]. 2017;4(2):2289-7577. Available from: http://publichealthmy.org/ejournal/ojs2/index.php/ijphcs/article/view/409

[7] Harmer M. Cancer of Breast. Bmj. 1955;1(4926):1391-1391.

[8] Arbyn M, Weiderpass E, Bruni L, de Sanjosé S, Saraiya M, Ferlay J, et al. Estimates of incidence and mortality of cervical cancer in 2018: a worldwide analysis. Lancet Glob Heal. 2020;8(2):e191–e203.

[9] Bosch FX, Lorincz A, Muñoz N, Meijer CJLM, Shah K V. The causal relation between human papillomavirus and cervical cancer. 2002;244-265.

[10] Schiffman M, Wentzensen N. Human papillomavirus (HPV) infection and the multi-stage carcinogenesis of cervical cancer Introduction and historic context. 2014;1854(4):1-14. Available from: https://www.ncbi.nlm.nih.gov/pmc/articles/PMC3711590/pdf/nihms-449612.pdf

[11] Flores R, Papenfuss M, Klimecki WT, Giuliano AR. Cross-sectional analysis of oncogenic HPV viral load and cervical intraepithelial neoplasia. 2006;1193(September 2005):1187-1193.

[12] Joharinia N, Farhadi A, Hosseini SY, Safaei A, Sarvari J. Association of HPV16 and 18 genomic copies with histological grades of cervical lesions. VirusDisease [Internet]. 2019;30(3):387-393. Available from: https://doi.org/10.1007/s13337-019-00545-2

[13] Mittal S, Basu P, Muwonge R, Banerjee D, Ghosh I, Sengupta MM. in high-risk HPV-positive women with normal cervix or. 2017;1859:1850-1859.

[14] Safaeian M, Schiffman M, Gage J, Solomon D, Wheeler CM, Castle PE. Detection of precancerous cervical lesions is differential by human papillomavirus type. Cancer Res. 2009;

Section 2

Screening

Chapter 3

The Role of AI in Cervical Cancer Screening

Bojana Turic, Xiaorong Sun, Jian Wang and Baochang Pang

Abstract

In the last few years internet-based technologies played an important role in reinventing various medical procedures and facilitating quick access to medical services and care, particularly in the remote areas of China. The use of artificial intelligence and cloud computing in clinical laboratory setting for slide analysis contributed to standardized cytology and pathology diagnosis but more importantly slide analysis with artificial intelligence has a huge potential to compensate for a country wide lack of pathologists and systematic quality control. While well-established automated slide scanning is already in use, we added intelligent algorithms located in a secure cloud for the better slide readings, and mobile phone microscopes to capture those regions of Hubei province where laboratory infrastructure is supported by high-speed internet and 5G networks. These technological advances allowed us to bring an important pathology expertise across the large areas of China.

Keywords: cervical cancer screening, artificial intelligence, cloud computing

1. Introduction

The contemporary artificial intelligence techniques such as machine learning applications were widely used in medicine and achieved the substantial success, particularly in radiology, in the recent years [1, 2]. Most of the technologies to support AI in pathology are still in development phase or are at the state of an observational study [3]. They are not widely applied in a large-scale screening as a routine service. This chapter will explain why and how AI and cloud computing is deployed as a standard of care in Province of Hubei, China and will illustrate all advantages that artificial intelligence can add making cervical cancer screening efficient and economically sound. This model can be easily adapted anywhere in the world where cytology is the only method or is combined with HPV in the cervical cancer screening.

2. Cervical cancer in China

In December 2020 China's National Health Commission (NHC) has voiced full support for the "Global Strategy to Accelerate the Elimination of Cervical Cancer" launched by the World Health Organization (WHO). According to data from 2018 cervical cancer is the fourth most frequent malignant tumor in women [4]. The same report shows that there were approximately 570000 cases of cervical cancer with estimated 310000 deaths globally. Peking University Health Care Center published that after 2000, the incidence of cervical cancer in China is on the rise while the mortality rate stayed somewhat the same. In 2015 the number of newly diagnosed cervical cancer cases was 98900 and the number of deaths reached 30500. However, in 2018 the reported number of cases were 106000 with 48000 deaths, which shows that the cervical cancer is indeed on the rise. That is particularly true for the women in rural areas. Since 2009, Chinese health authorities initiated free large-scale population-based cervical cancer screening for rural women with low socioeconomic status totaling approximately 10 million people [5]. These early initiatives were important and laid the foundation for cervical cytology screening guideline development in China. It is fair to say that these early initiatives were also important for bringing awareness about the importance of cervical examination among women.

3. How cervical cancer screening methodology was introduced?

Detecting cervical precancerous lesions and implementing early screening followed by early treatment intervention are proven essential steps in prevention and treatment of cervical cancer. Decrease in cervical cancer incidence in most western countries can be attributed to the success of screening using the Papanicolaou test (PAP-test) where this method has proved to effectively reduce cervical cancer incidence and mortality [6, 7]. PAP-test is based on detecting cellular changes that can progress into malignant changes but if detected at an early stage can be treated and prevent development of cervical cancer. It has been shown in many countries around the world that implementing PAP-test in systematic, comprehensive screening programs can reduce incidence of cervical cancer. In recent years, HPV-DNA virus examination methods have also been introduced into cervical cancer screening [8]. The success and program implementation differ among countries and so in China too, in certain areas it is introduced with questionable success. In the western countries for example in Canada and Japan, more traditional cytology analysis methods are still used [9], while UK, USA and Australia use HPV detection methods [10–12].

4. Why is AI and cloud computing the best approach for mass screening?

Due to China's huge and growing population, a simple "mirror" of the European or American guidelines for cervical screening is not possible due to several major differences in the medical system organization: (1) In China, the primary point of sample collection is not a family physician office setting like in the most of the western countries, but gynecologist, or specially trained nurse (2) There is an insufficient number of laboratory professionals, particularly cytotechnicians to screen, read the slides and issue negative reports and (3) Organized quality control and assurance is not established nationwide and it varies from laboratory to laboratory. The lack of cytotechicians and cytopathologists in county's and town's level medical institutions make cervical cancer screening uneven thus in many places, the purpose of screening is lost [13].

In the recent years we saw rapid development in deep learning and artificial intelligence technologies. The intelligent recognition of medical images and counting method of deep learning has made possible the use of the artificial intelligence (AI) in diagnostic techniques such as X-ray, CT, mammography and pathology [14–17]. With the data quality and improvements of speed in automated microscopes and whole slide scanners [18], telepathology was introduced as a first step for remote slide interpretation [19]. The adoption was slow however today telepathology is an integral part of almost every pathology laboratory particularly for second opinion. It was logical that the next technological development, the use of artificial intelligence in laboratory medicine came after years of research and systems training with millions of cervical specimens.

The first AI diagnostic techniques for use in a large-scale cervical cancer screening in primary hospitals without cytopathologists was implemented in Hubei province, China. It allowed diagnosis without physical transportation of samples (slides); data are analyzed in the cloud at the very high speed. When AI was introduced (2017) it greatly reduced the financial, time cost and improved the accessibility of expert pathologist and fast turnaround for cytology results to patients [20]. These were the first steps towards today's use of AI for slide scanning and robotic data analysis. Furthermore, today we do not even need the fully developed scanner, the new mobile phone microscopes particularly in the remote and rural areas are used and are already improving the way cervical cancer screening is delivered.

5. The start of AI and cloud computing in cervical cancer screening, Hubei Province, China

In 2017, Hubei's Provincial Health Authority authorized a cervical cancer screening program that used a unique cloud-based platform for cervical cancer screening, data gathering, analysis, review and reporting to provide screening services to rural women in the province. The project was authorized by Ethic Review Board who agreed to approve the project. Data were continuously collected and presented for a final authorization to use AI as a standard in a cervical cancer screening.

From January 1, 2018 to December 31, 2018, a total of 703,103 women were screened for cervical cancer and those data are published recently (**Figure 1**). The vast majority were women between 30 and 65 years of age. Out of the total number of women 30,035 (4.3%) were between the ages of 20 and 30, and 8,313 (1.2%) were over 65 years of age. All women were of low socioeconomic status and from 83 counties in China's Hubei Province. As mentioned earlier the objective of the program was to assess the feasibility of a cloud-based screening program and the management of healthcare statistics.

Without going into too many details, which are published elsewhere [21], our study showed high agreement rate for normal cytology grade between AI and manual reading. We showed that well-"trained AI system" can accurately classify normal cytology. In our case more than 99% of women classified as normal cytology by AI were confirmed by manual reading, suggesting that most of women with normal cytology could be primarily excluded by AI. In other words, AI system identified majority of slides most likely to be normal as only needing rapid review. This was a very important finding for laboratories that handle over 1 million slides in a short period.

AI-assisted cytology showed increased sensitivity without substantial decrease in specificity for detection of CIN2+, compared with manual reading, in accordant with previous observational studies using automated cytology [18, 19]. In our study, the detection of histological CIN2+ among women classified as normal by manual reading and abnormal by AI, was substantially higher than that among women classified as normal by AI and abnormal by manual reading. The detection of CIN2+ in our study was higher than the national program (155 versus 125 per 100 000), which can perhaps be explained because all women were from rural areas whose incidence is higher than countries average.

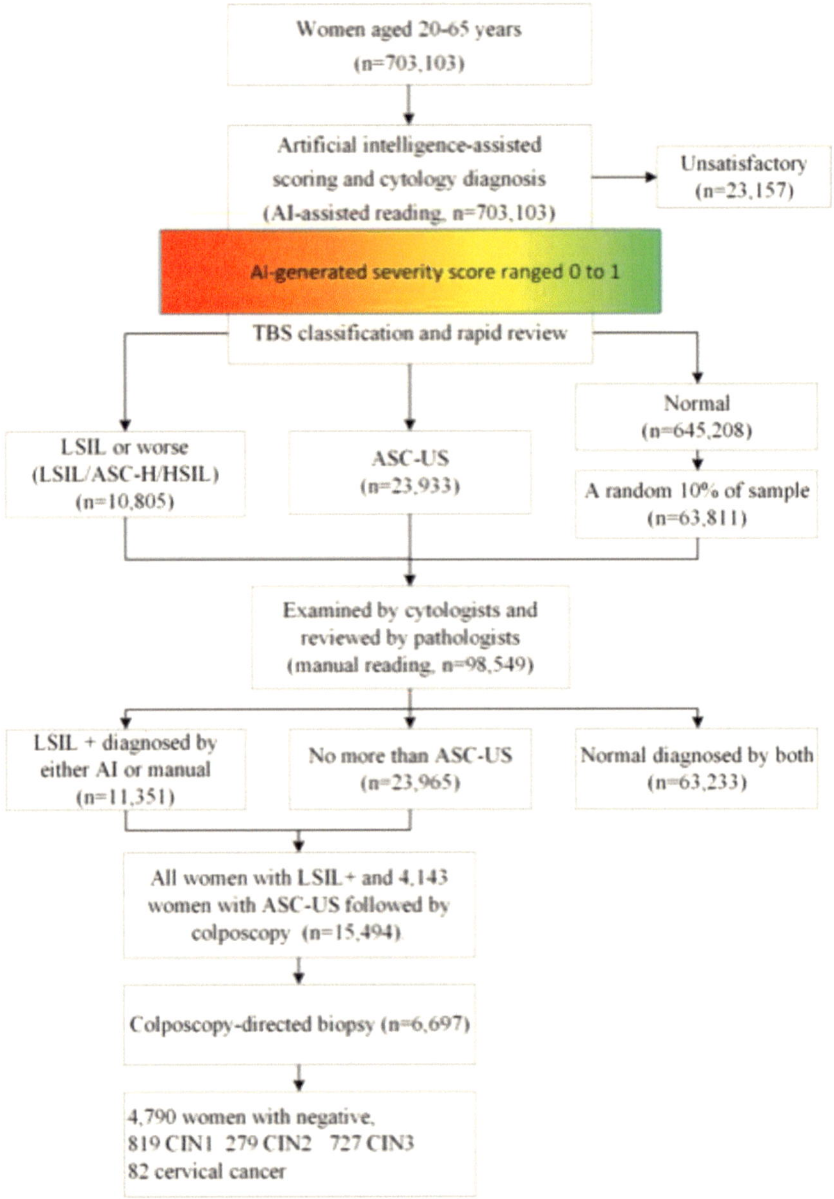

Figure 1.
The main study flow and the points at which data were collected.

An important issue of cytology-based cervical cancer screening is the management of women with ASC-US, in which detection of high-grade lesions or cancer varies greatly. Inappropriate triage may result in an over referral of colposcopy, or a delayed diagnosis and treatment. Although human papillomavirus test, genotyping or some biomarkers (e.g. methylation, p16/Ki-67) provide technology for triaging ASC-US, these algorithms are very limited in low-resource settings.

AI-assisted cytology system provides opportunities to address many difficulties that cervical cancer screening in China is facing. In the mode of AI-assisted cytology-based cervical cancer screening, large number of slides are automatically scanned and transferred to electronic cytology images and classified by pre-trained deep learning algorithms. For example, our laboratory received over 2 million slides in 2019. Although the system is automated each abnormal (positive) slide is still reviewed by cytologists who can log in into the cloud and review remotely and randomly selected 10% negative for quality control purposes.

Although the performance of automated-assisted cytology reading as a primary screening was reported previously [22] to our best knowledge, our study was the largest scale population-based cervical cancer screening using AI-assisted cytology reading in the low- and middle-income countries followed by AI routine implementation for cervical cancer screening. Once data were presented to our health authorities, we were allowed to offer cervical cancer screening based on AI as a routine clinical service.

6. Current implementation

Landing complete AI system has three major key components: an automated slide scanner installed in laboratories of counites hospitals, data uploading, and cloud platform for data processing and storing. The cloud system also connects to end users (physicians and patients) providing them with test reports (patients receive only negative report directly on their cell phone). See **Figure 2**.

The system is continuously improved due to the increasing participation in large-scale cervical cancer screening activities and therefore database is growing exponentially. For example, parallel to our study in 2018, we performed additional analysis of more than 1.2 million cell samples, adding millions of microscopic images to database. With increasing data, the algorithm is also upgraded and improved, leading to improved diagnosis and detection rates of cervical abnormalities.

In response to the need for timely reporting and analysis of massive data from dispersed areas, Landing has improved its data uploading and downloading efficiencies. Data processing capacity of our "Cyto Cloud" is increased from processing 30 million cell samples per day in the end of 2016 to 750 million per day by the end of 2018.

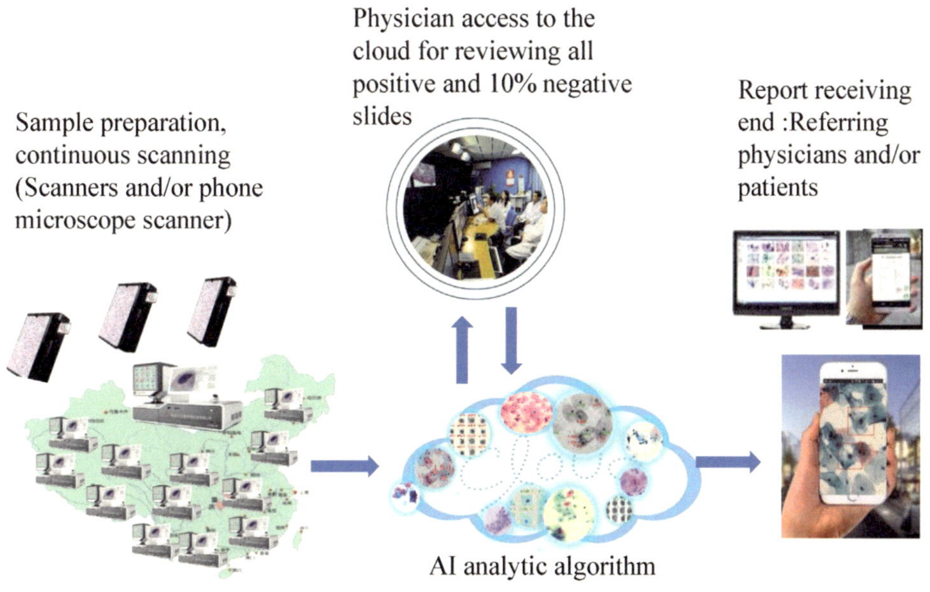

Figure 2.
Operational steps within cervical cancer screening program.

This mode is being proved to be practical in China and can be reproducible in other developing countries wherever cytology is used as only method or is combined with HPV testing. Moreover, technological advancements and data accumulation might enable the AI system to be more intelligent and used more generally in other diagnostic fields.

7. Conclusions

Further development of AI and cloud computing in laboratory medicine is inevitable. Once huge amount of data is collected and analyzed the basic unit of data collection is now ready for a new roll out. In collaboration with a mobile phone companies the next generation of automated scanners is in the form of handheld phone microscopes that can be used in a remote area without lot of infrastructure. (Landing Smart Hand held device) It is important to say that the mobile phone handheld microscope is not only limited for the use in the cervical cancer screening. It is and can be used for any cytology and/or histology slides. While cervical cancers samples are currently the only specimens that use AI for assisted analysis the handheld device can be used for assisted second opinion diagnosis of FNA or bronchial washings or any other type of cytology or histology slides.

AI, fast cloud computing through 5G networks is changing the way we deliver medicine today. These advances are offering tremendous opportunity for improvement of screening programs, particularly in China where huge number of women need to be screened. At the same time our model can be easily applicable, adaptable and implemented anywhere in the world where there is a lack of laboratory professionals and there is a need for a cervical cancer screening improvement.

Conflict of interest

The authors declare no conflict of interest.

Author details

Bojana Turic*, Xiaorong Sun, Jian Wang and Baochang Pang
Landing Medical High Tech Co., Wuhan, China

*Address all correspondence to: bojana.turic@gmail.com

References

[1] Hosny A, Parmar C, Quackenbush J, Schwartz LH, Aerts HJWL. Artificial intelligence in radiology. Nat Rev Cancer. 2018;18(8):500-510. doi:10.1038/s41568-018-0016-5

[2] Oren O, Gersh B, Bhatt D, Artificial intelligence in medical imaging; switching from radiographic pathological data to clinically meaningful endpoints The Lancet Digital Health 2020;vol 2(9):486-488. doi.org/10.1016/S2589-7500(20) 30160-6

[3] Hu L, Bell D, Antani S, et al. An Observational Study of Deep Learning and Automated Evaluation of Cervical Images for Cancer Screening. J Natl Cancer Inst. 2019;111(9):923-932. doi:10.1093/jnci/djy225

[4] Arbyn M, Weiderpass E, Bruni L, Sanjosé S, Saraiya M, Ferlay J, Bray F ; Estimates of incidence and mortality of cervical cancer in 2018: a worldwide analysis The Lancet Global Health,2020; vol 8(2):191-203/doi.org/10.1016/ S2214-109X(19)30482-6

[5] Li J., Kang L., Qiao Y.: Review of the Cervical Cancer Disease Burden in Mainland China, Asian Pacific J Cancer Prev, 12, 1149-1153

[6] Cohen PA, Cervical Cancer, Lancet, 2019, 393,169-182.

[7] Wang Y, Wei L, Liu J, Li S, Wang Q, Comparison of Cancer Incidence between China and the USA Cancer Biol Med 2012; 9: 128-132 doi: 10.3969/j

[8] Dickinson JA, Stankiewic A, Popadiuk C, et al. Reduced cervical cancer incidence and mortality in Canada: national data from 1932 to 2006. BMC public health. 2012, 12:992

[9] Hamashima C., Aoki D., Miyagi E., et al., The Japanese Guideline for Cervical Cancer Screening, Jpn J Clin Oncol 2010 40(6)485-502

[10] NHS Cervical Screening Program 2016 NHSCSP Publication number 20

[11] US Preventive Service Task Force: Screening for Cervical Cancer JAMA. 2018;320(7):674-686

[12] Australian Institute of Health and Welfare: Cervical Cancer screening 2018

[13] Di J. Rutherford S., Chu C.: Review of the Cervical Cancer Burden and Population-Based Cervical Cancer Screening in China, Asian Pac J Cancer Prev., 2015 16 (17), 7401-740711.

[14] Wang L. Alexander C : Medical Application and Healthcare Based on Cloud Computing International Journal of Cloud Computing and Services Science (IJ-CLOSER) Vol.2, No.4, August 2014, pp. 217~225

[15] Lau J., Lehnert E., Sethi A., et al. The Cancer Genomics Cloud: Collaborative, Reproducible, and Democratized—A New Paradigm in Large-Scale Computational Research Cancer Res; 77(21) November 1, 2017

[16] Yang C., Huang Q., Li Z., Liu K., Hu F. Big Data and cloud computing: innovation opportunities and challenges, International Journal of Digital Earth, 2017 10:1, 13-53

[17] Moreno P, Joly Y, Knoppers B Public-Private Partnership in Cloud–Computing Services in the Context of Genomic Frontiers in Medicine 20 January 2017

[18] Wu M, Yan C, Liu H, Liu Q, Yin Y. Automatic classification of cervical cancer from cytological images by using convolutional neural network. Biosci Rep. 2018 Nov 28;38(6):BSR20181769. doi: 10.1042/BSR20181769. Erratum in:

Biosci Rep. 2019 Apr 2;39(4): PMID: 30341239; PMCID: PMC6259017.

[19] Evans AJ, Salama ME, Henricks WH, Pantanowitz L. Implementation of Whole Slide Imaging for Clinical Purposes: Issues to Consider From the Perspective of Early Adopters. Arch Pathol Lab Med. 2017 Jul;141(7):944-959. doi: 10.5858/arpa.2016-0074-OA. Epub 2017 Apr 25. PMID: 28440660.

[20] Dong Y, Bai J, Zhang Y , Shang G, Zhao Y , Li S , Yan N , Hao S, Zhang W, Automated Quantitative Cytology Imaging Analysis System in Cervical Cancer Screening in Shanxi Province, China Cancer and Clinical Oncology; 2017, Vol. 6 (2); ISSN 1927-4858 E-ISSN 1927-4866 doi:10.5539/cco.v6n2p51

[21] Bao H, Sun X, Zhang Y, Pang B, Li H, Zhou L, Wu F, Cao D, Wang J, Turic B, Wang L. The artificial intelligence-assisted cytology diagnostic system in large-scale cervical cancer screening: A population-based cohort study of 0.7 million women. Cancer Med. 2020 Sep;9(18):6896-6906. doi: 10.1002/cam4.3296. Epub 2020 Jul 22. PMID: 32697872; PMCID: .

[22] Hu L, Bell D, Antani S, Xue Z, Yu K, Horning MP, Gachuhi N, Wilson B, Jaiswal MS, Befano B, Long LR, Herrero R, Einstein MH, Burk RD, Demarco M, Gage JC, Rodriguez AC, Wentzensen N, Schiffman M. An Observational Study of Deep Learning and Automated Evaluation of Cervical Images for Cancer Screening. J Natl Cancer Inst. 2019 Sep 1;111(9):923-932. doi: 10.1093/jnci/djy225. PMID: 30629194; PMCID: PMC6748814.

Chapter 4

The Presence of HPV in Dental Calculus: It's Role in Pathogenesis of Oral and Cervical Cancer

Sunardhi Widyaputra, Natallia Pranata, Ignatius Setiawan and Jamas Ari Anggraini

Abstract

Human papillomavirus (HPV) infection accounts for approximately 5.2% of the worldwide human cancer burden. Molecular epidemiologic evidence clearly indicates that certain types of HPV are the principal cause of both cervical and oral cancers. Major oncoproteins E6 and E7 can inactivate p53 and pRB proteins because it happened genome instability and dysregulation host cell cycles. This virus is an epithelial tropism, vulnerable area mainly at the basal layer and epithelial stem cell, because it still has a high proliferation capacity, so it can support the replication of the virus. Virions bind initially to the glycosaminoglycan (GAG) chains of heparan sulphate proteoglycan (HSPG). More than 99% cervical cancer arise at the cervical transformation zone. In oral cavity, exposed areas of the basal layer will be very susceptible to HPV infection. The HPV presence in the oral area is considered as one of the etiologics of oral cancer in those who do not have bad habits such as smoking, betel chewing, or poor oral hygiene. Our study successfully identified HPV type 58 in dental calculus. Dental calculus, calcified oral plaque biofilm, has been shown to be an abundant, nearly ubiquitous, and long-term reservoir of the ancient oral microbiome, including bacteria, archaea, eukaryote, and viruses. During biomineral maturation process, several biological contents around the oral region should be trapped, including the exfoliated virus contained cells. Dental calculus is a promising source of HPV and carcinogens molecules in the oral cavity and could be used as a biomarker for early detection.

Keywords: HPV, biosource, dental calculus, oral cancer, cervical cancer, OSCC

1. Introduction

Human papillomavirus (HPV) is considered to be one of the oldest known viruses and also the most common sexually transmitted infection (STI). Annually, around 6 million people are diagnosed with the disease [1]. HPV-related diseases have been an important subject to study for many years and are becoming a major concern for public health at present [2, 3]. This virus is an epithelial tropism, a vulnerable area mainly at the basal layer and epithelial stem cells [3]. After infecting cells, HPV will change the cellular environment, avoiding the immune response, so that the infection can persist [4]. This virus is very varied, there are about 228 genotypes that live in the human body [5]. If HPVs have 70% similarity in the DNA sequence, they are categorized as belonging to the same genus [3]. Alphapapillomavirus is a genus which mainly infects the mucosa both in the anogenital tract and in the oral cavity [3, 6]. HPV was confirmed to cause cervical cancer in early 1980s. It is estimated that around 70% of head and neck cancer cases are also caused by HPV infection of the genus alpha [6, 7]. Based on its role in carcinogenesis, HPV is divided into high risk (HR) and low risk (LR). LR-HPV such as HPV-6 and HPV-11 cause benign papilloma/condyloma, whereas HR-HPV such as HPV-16 and HPV-18 cause squamous intraepithelial lesions that can develop into squamous cell carcinoma [8].

A significant change in HPV endemic is indicated in the epidemiological data from the last decade. HPV is not only found in the genital area but also in the oral area [7, 9]. HPV infection in the oral cavity is frequently associated with sexual behavior. Oral sex is considered a risky sexual behavior that has the potential to transmit HPV from the anogenital to the oral cavity [10].

This chapter aims to describe the causality of HPV infection in the oral cavity and in the genital area, especially the causes of "endemic" triggered by changes in the behavior of the society. Knowledge of the history of HPV infection, risk factors, clinical manifestations, current prevention, and therapy strategies is indispensable prerequisite for health workers to improve the professionalism of dentists and other medical personnel involved in treating patients at risk of infection or patients with clinical risk manifestations of infection.

Since HPV infection is latent, to be able to study the pathogenesis of HPV-linked oral cancer, it is necessary to have a biosource that can detect the presence of the causative agent for a long time [7]. Dental calculus, as a biosource, can keep a variety of molecular information, including HPV DNA, for a long time [11]. Therefore, it is imperative to design sufficient prevention and management strategies to tackle HPV-related diseases, while promoting understanding and collaboration among health workers: the medical and dental communities, who may not yet familiarize themselves with this perspective.

2. Pathogenesis of HPV infections and cervical cancer

HPV is a small double-stranded circular DNA virus that commonly infects humans [12, 13]. HPV is almost entirely acquired from sexual exposure, when it enters the skin and mucous membranes of the mouth, anus, penis, and female reproductive tract [14]. Infections with different strains are linked to a variety of skin manifestations, ranging from common warts to malignancies [15]. HPV infection accounts for approximately 5.2% of human cancer burden worldwide, including the cancers of the anus, genital tract, and oropharynx [16].

2.1 Characteristics of HPV

HPV is a heterogeneous viral group of the papillomaviridae family that infects the basal layer of either the vertebrates mucosal epithelial or cutaneous, causes neoplasia, or persists without symptoms [17]. HPV contains a double-stranded circular non-enveloped DNA genome that codes for eight genes and a noncoding region that manages a replication of the viral and controls cellular and transcription of the viral [16, 18]. All protein-coding genes are located on the same DNA strand. The genes are divided into early (E) and late (L) genes, E1, E2, E4,E5, E6, E7, L1, and L2, with the late genes encoding the major and minor capsid proteins [18, 19]. The capsid is the protein shell that surrounds the viral DNA. HPV can integrate into the host cell chromosomes and/or persist in episomal form [20].

One of important factor in HPV-related diseases is epigenetic regulation of viral gene expression [21, 22]. Another investigation is that the viral genome can be methylated de novo by host DNA methyltransferase (DNMT), implying an innate response to pathogens [23]. Thus methylation of the viral genome may be in part a mechanism by which the host attempts to suppress viral gene expression and thereby HPV pathogenicity [21].

HPV are characterized according to their tissue tropism and they are subdivided into five main genera (Alpha-, beta-, gamma-, nu- and mu-papillomaviruses) depending on the DNA sequences, HPV life cycle characteristics and disease associations [24]. Traditionally HPV is distinguished, based on the tropicalism of specific epithelium, on the skin type and mucosa: the first infects the skin of the hands and feet, the second prefers the mucosal surface of the upper gastrointestinal tract, the anogenital area, the urethra and conjunctive [25]. The HPV can be further subdivided according to the epidemiological classification as ones with low and high risk oncogenic potentials depending on the viruses' ability to promote the proliferation of infected cells and lead to malignant transformations [26]. HR-HPV is associated with an increased risk of developing cancer and is often referred to as a 'cancer related' or 'oncogenic' type [27]. This group has HPV genotypes such as 16–18–31-33-35, 39,45,51,52,53, 56,58,59, 66, 67,70,73,68, 82) [28]. HR-HPV is associated with potentially and obviously malignant lesions (e.g. anogenital cancer) [3]. LR-HPV has genotypes such as 2, 4, 27 (skin type) and mucosal types 6, 11, 13, 32, 42) [28]. LR-HPV is more commonly associated with non-malignant diseases (e.g. ordinary warts, condyloma, focal epithelial hyperplasia, squamous cell papilloma) [29].

2.2 Effect of HPV on the basal layer and epithelial stem cells

Papillomavirus infections are usually long-lived and persistent and the dividing basal cells must provide a continual reservoir of infected cells for the overlying virus producing tissue [30]. Thus, HPV need a robust mechanism to retain their episomal genomes within the nucleus of dividing epithelial cells [31]. In normal squamous epithelium of the cervix, the basal layer is the area of active cell division [14]. After division, the cells migrate up from the basal layer and no longer progress through the cell cycle and become terminally differentiated keratinocytes [32]. Since epithelial cells have stopped dividing at this stage, the number of virus copies per cell has increased considerably and the level of viral gene expression has also increased [14]. Most of the replication of the viral genome occurs after epithelial cells are shed from the basal layer [32]. The histopathological changes characteristic of typical low-grade HPV-induced lesions reflect active replication of the virus [14]. These include koilocytosis, multinucleation, and nuclear enlargement and are due to the assembly of the viral particles in the upper epithelial layers [30]. The epithelium is then shed, and infectious HPV virions are released, which can then infect a new host [31].

New insights have identified the capacity for HPV early region genes to dysregulate adult tissue stem cell self-renewal pathways ensuring that the expanded population preserve its stem cell characteristics beyond the stem cell niche. HPV-infected cells acquire additional transforming mutations that can give rise to intraepithelial neoplasia (IEN), from environmental factors such as sunlight or tobacco induced mutations in skin and oral cavity, respectively. With establishment of IEN, HPV viral replication is sacrificed with loss of the episome, and the tissue is predisposed to multiple cancer stem cell-driven carcinomas [33].

2.3 HPV and the potential for malignancy

Recent molecular and epidemiological studies showed HPV infection is now a well-established cause of cervical cancer and there is growing evidence of HPV being a relevant factor in other anogenital cancers (anus, vulva, vagina and penis) as well as head and neck cancers [34, 35]. Kian Ang's research (2010) suggested the role of HPV infection in the pathogenesis of oropharyngeal cancer; 63,8% of patients with oropharyngeal cancer (206 of 323) were HPV-positive [36].

HPV-induced carcinogenesis occurs as a multi-step process [16]. It begins by primary infection of the proliferating basal cells of the squamous epithelium [32]. If the infection is caused by a HR-HPV type, and there are presence of failure of the immune system to control and clear the infection plus the presence of some co-factors, after a period of time, HPV infection continues to accumulate sufficient genomic instability and leads to epithelial neoplastic transformation [18]. HPV is carcinogenic, partly because proteins E6 and E7 cause abnormal regulation of p53 and Rb, control of apoptosis and regulation of cell cycle [37]. It is believed that the circular genome is linearized and integrated as a late event in the infection process, destroying the region of the E1/E2 gene, destroying the E2 gene, releasing the suppression of the viral genome, leading to the overexpression of E6 viruses and E7 genes to maintain the malignant phenotype [38]. E5, E6 and E7 proteins are the most important for oncogenic transformation [39]. In the early stages of carcinogenesis the E5 protein plays a role and appears to increase cellular EGFR signaling, leading to up-regulation of viral gene expression and cell proliferation [37]. Generally, the high-risk HPV E6 protein activates many cellular proteins, including the cellular ubiquitin ligase E6AP, which targets the degradation of the TP53 protein, leading to loss of TP53-mediated processes, including apoptosis mediated by TP53 and the cell cycle checkpoints, DNA damage response and chromosome stability [19, 40]. Low risk E6 will not degrade TP53 [19]. The E7 protein promotes the proliferation of HPV-infected cells by degrading the RB1 protein, releasing E2F transcription factors, and boosting the expression of S-phase cell cycle genes and their proteins (including CDKN2A and its protein p16INK4a) [41]. This protein can be used as a surrogate marker for HPV expression [42]. The expression of E6 and E7 genes not only eliminates the two most important cellular tumor suppressor pathways, namely RB1 and TP53, but also affects the expression of a variety of tumor suppressor genes, DNA damage response genes and oncogenes, resulting in carcinogenic transformation [41].

3. HPV in the oral cavity

In oral cavity, exposed areas of the basal layer will be very susceptible to HPV infection. The presence of HPV in the oral cavity is thought to be the etiologic of oral cancer in those who do not have bad habits such as smoking, betel chewing or poor oral hygiene.

3.1 Characteristics of oral microbiome

Microbiome is the community of microbial residents in our body. It is the ecological community of symbiotic, commensal, and pathogenic microorganisms [43]. The human microbiome defines either the microorganisms (bacteria, archaea, lower and higher eukaryotes, and viruses) found in and on the human body or their collective genomes. The microbiota takes part in regulating the immune response, affecting the appetite, and therefore changing the food intake pattern, participating in vitamin biosynthesis, and protecting human beings by producing antimicrobial substances [44].

The gut microbiome has been most extensively studied, however, microorganisms actually inhabit all the barrier surfaces of the human body including the skin, the oral cavity, the nasopharynx, the esophagus and stomach, and also the vagina, the urinary tract, the lungs and others. The composition of the microbiome varies according to the anatomic site. Different individuals have different compositions of microbiome [45]. The most common reproducible microbiome archetypes, or community-state types (CSTs) found in cervical intraepithelial neoplasia (CIN) patients are CSTs characterized by Lactobacillus depletion, anaerobic bacteria predominance, and Lactobacillus iners dominance. These CSTs are significantly associated with preinvasive diseases, increased disease severity, and disease invasiveness [46]. *L. crispatus*, L. iners, and ureaplasma parvum are associated with the pro-inflammatory inflammasome molecules IL-1α and IL-18, concomitantly with the antagonist IL-1ra generating a balance between anti-inflammatory and pro-inflammatory responses. This equilibrium is imbalanced by the presence of pathogens, which diverts it toward the inflammation [47].

Oral microbiome is defined as the collective genome of microorganisms that live in the oral cavity. After the gut, the oral cavity is the second largest microbial community in humans [43]. The oral cavity of healthy individuals contains hundreds of different bacterial, viral, and fungal species. Many of these can join to form biofilms which are resistant to mechanical stress or antibiotic treatment. Most are also commensal species, however, they can become pathogenic when triggered by changes in the environment or in the oral cavity, including changes in the quality of an individual's personal hygiene.

Those microorganisms can have very dynamic behavior, adapting to a wide range of environments and interactions with other microbial species in biofilms. The formation of biofilms may occur on many kinds of surfaces in the oral cavity. The epithelial cells, saliva-coated enamel, dental surfaces, primary colonizing bacteria, and orthodontics together provide suitable environments for the establishment of mixed-species biofilms [48]. Most organisms can only survive in the oropharynx when they stick to either the soft tissues or the hard surfaces. Otherwise, they may be removed by swallowing and chewing movements, nose blowing force, tongue movements and oral hygiene implements, the wash-out effect of the saliva, nasal and crevicular fluid outflow, and the active motion of the cilia of the nasal and sinus walls [49].

The oral cavity has three different sites, including mucosal surfaces, hard tissues, and exocrine gland tissue, all of which present unique characteristics for microbiota composition. The tongue, the gingiva, the buccal mucosa, and the palate are mucosal surfaces, while the teeth are hard tissues in the oral cavity [44]. Based on their anatomical location there are different oral mucosal surfaces. The oral mucosa surfaces, in general, can be divided into masticatory and non-masticatory mucosa. The attached gingiva around the teeth, the hard palate, and the upper surface of the tongue are the masticatory mucosa, which also known as keratinized stratified squamous epithelium. The taste buds of the lingual papillae are found on the upper surface of the tongue. The rest of the oral cavity including buccal and labial sites, as well as at the floor of the mouth are non-masticatory mucosa or stratified squamous nonkeratinized epithelium. Teeth are hard structures, which are in contact closely with mucosa in the oral cavity. There is no structure in the human body like the condition of the oral cavity. In the oral cavity there is also the gingival sulcus, which is located between the teeth and the mucosal gingiva, is an important anatomical site for the formation of dental plaque biofilm [44].

Saliva also has an important role in oral health. Saliva is excreted by the major and minor salivary glands. The main salivary gland openings are located at the floor of the mouth, the caruncles sublingual, while those in the buccal mucosa are called the Stensen's duct. About 1–2 L/day of saliva is naturally produced and swallowed. Saliva is fundamentally composed of water, electrolytes, mucus, antibacterial material, and enzymes that help to process food and kill bacteria. Saliva has very essential function in maintain oral health. The prevalence of oral diseases, such as dental caries, gingivitis, and periodontitis, increments fundamentally without saliva [44].

The total volume of oral microbial is around 1011 microbes/mL. The primary type of microbial found in the oral cavity is Streptococcus. The others are Leptotrichia, Porphyromonas, Veillonella, Prevotella, Haemophilus, Propionibacterium, Staphylococcus, and Treponema [44]. There is a symbiotic relationship among the microorganisms in the oral cavity to gain mutual benefits. The commensal populations are harmless and maintain a check on the pathogenic species by not allowing them to adhere to the mucosa. The bacteria become pathogenic only after they breach the barrier of the commensals, causing infection and disease [43].

Oral microbiome profiles from both healthy controls and HPV-negative oral cavity cancer (OCC) and oropharyngeal cancer (OPC) patients suggested that the presence of HPV affected the composition of the oral microbiome [46]. HPV-positive OCC and OPC patients both showed an abundance of Gemella and Leuconostoc, while Haemophilus correlated with HPV infection. The 16S rRNA sequencing on saliva and oral rinse samples of OCC and OPC patients showed a decrease in richness and diversity when compared to control patients. This decrease in diversity was opposite the case of cervical patients and indicated that a few dominating, pathogenic bacteria might have influence on HPV persistence and carcinogenesis in the oral environment [46]. Interestingly, Lactobacillus spp. were found to be significantly associated with the saliva samples from HPV-positive OPC patients [3, 50]. In a follow-up study, species-level context was provided for the Lactobacillus spp. using high-resolution 16S rRNA analysis. A subset of OPC patient samples were enriched with commensal species from the vaginal flora, including L. gasseri/johnsonii and *L. vaginalis*. This was not observed in control groups nor in the saliva from the Human Microbiome Project [51]. This suggested that these normally commensal vaginal species could have been transferred to the oral flora during oral sex, which, if validated, would have interesting implications in the role of vaginal-associated Lactobacillus in oral HPV disease.

3.2 Correlation between oral microbiome, chronic inflammation, and HPV infection

As part of the digestive tract, the oral cavity has diverse microorganisms and oral microbiota is a complex microbial community. The oral microbiota plays an important role in human health, and dysbiosis of oral microbiota can induce many kinds of local and systemic diseases [50]. In this dysbiosis of oral microbiota, the host's immune system will be stimulated by the inflammatory process. If this condition persists, the inflammation will become chronic [52]. Chronic inflammation occurs the most frequently in tooth supporting tissues [53]. The average prevalence of periodontitis in the general population is 30% [54].

Periodontitis is an advanced gingival disease induced by dysbiosis of bacterial and it can eventually result in tooth missing. It begins as gingival bleeding in response to inflammation, after that bacterial biofilm accumulates around the tooth cervical surfaces [44, 49]. The damage continues to spread to the periodontal tissue. There is a migration of the junctional epithelium toward the apical, the gum groove becomes more than 3 mm deep, which is called the periodontal pocket. In the connective tissues, there is an increase in angiogenesis, chronic inflammatory infiltrates, fibrosis, loss of connective tissues, clinical attachment loss (CAL) and resorption of the alveolar bones/alveolar bone loss (ABL) [55].

Risk factors for oral and pharyngeal cancers are age, tobacco use, frequent use of alcohol, and exposure to sunlight. A higher incidence of cancer development is also found in individuals with chronic inflammatory conditions. An increased risk of developing oral squamous cell carcinoma (OSCC) associated with periodontitis suggests a possible role of inflammation caused by the microbiome with oral cancer. Periodontitis is a typical example of an infectious disease causing chronic inflammation in the oral cavity [56]. Recent evidence proved the role of microbiome-derived signals in the pathogenesis of several chronic inflammatory diseases. Periodontal diseases have been associated with the risk for precancerous lesions, tumors, and oral neoplasms. The third National Health and Nutrition Examination Survey (NHANES III) discovered that periodontitis was significantly related to HPV status in patients with oropharyngeal cancer [49].

Well-known periodontal pathogens, such as Tannerella forsythia, Porphyromonas gingivalis (P. gingivalis), and Treponema denticola, are not usually detected in the oral cavities of healthy human beings [44]. Oral bacteria could affect the outcome of viral infection. This is evident in the case of P. gingivalis, which upregulates expression of CCR5 [48]. P. gingivalis also causes the expression of the B7-H1 and B7-DC receptors in primary OSCC, which are upregulated in a variety of cancers and contribute to chronic inflammation [57].

Chronic infection with P. gingivalis and Fusobacterium nucleatum has been recently demonstrated to promote tongue tumors in a murine model through direct interaction with oral epithelial cells, leading to upregulation of the IL-6-STAT3 pathway in a TLR2-dependent manner [56]. P. gingivalis was also shown to cause gingival epithelial cells (GECs) to migrate in a manner which depends on the overexpression of Zeb1, an activator of the epithelial-mesenchymal transition (EMT). Moreover, P. gingivalis increases proliferation and promotes invasion and migration in an in vitro model of persistent infection. Furthermore, P. gingivalis infection hinders the activity of glycogen synthase kinase 3 (GSK3b), an important EMT regulator, in primary oral epithelial cells. In addition, other EMT-associated transcription factors, as well as mesenchymal intermediates, such as vimentin, MMP-2, MMP-7, and MMP-9, increase and are associated with higher levels of cell migration [58].

Expression of pro-inflammatory cytokines in periodontal disease such as IL-1 and TNF-a has been related to microbial triggered carcinogenesis [59]. In a study comparing the microbiome of gingival squamous cell carcinoma (GSCC) with periodontitis microbiome, members of the genera Fusobacterium, Peptostreptococcus, and Prevotella were found more abundant in cancerous, periodontal tissues. In contrast, saliva or soft mucosa concealed more periodontal health-related bacteria [60].

What shall we do to minimize diseases caused by the oral microbiota? The most obvious recommendation is to improve oral hygiene; however, people with sufficient oral hygiene can still develop chronic infections due to the composition of resident microbiota and changes in the host's immune response.

3.3 Transmission of oral HPV infection

Most HPV transmission is thought to occur as a result of microscopic mucosal erosion during sexual activity [61, 62]. HPV can cause latent infection in basal cells after mucosal epithelial surface erosion by low HPV DNA copy; transmission of infection can occur only when the number of the viruses is sufficient [63].

HPV can also cause subclinical infection that is active but asymptomatic; or clinical infection leading to benign, potentially malignant or malignant lesions [39, 63]. Most HPV infections are cleared by the immune system; the individual is not aware he or she has had the infection and does not develop visible lesions or cancer [64, 65].

Unlike many viruses, HPV requires the infected cells to divide and differentiate. The epidermis is composed of multiple keratinocyte layers, and is the component that papillomaviruses target [3]. HPV infection starts when the viruses enter epithelial basal cells which are referred to as the target cells of the virus [32]. HPV binds epithelial cell heparin sulfate proteoglycans and cell specific receptors to gain entry by both clathrin-dependent and -independent endocytosis [66]. Infection leads to the establishment of the HPV circular double-stranded genome as a stable episome within some cells of the basal layer [67]. In the case of alpha-HPV, the viral genome can integrate into the host genome, whereas for beta-HPV, the viral genome remains episomal [68].

After entering the host cell, HPV infection can manifest in two clinical circumstances: 1) Subclinical or invisible infection, i.e. the tacit presence of the viral genome to the inoculation site without clinical and/or histological and/or cytologic changes in the cervical mucosa; 2) clinical infections, expression of proliferation of infected keratinocytes and associated with clinical and histological lesions of the cervical mucosa [69–71]. These lesions are usually benign when the infection is sustained by LR-HPV [72]. Otherwise HR-HPV infection, especially when settled for more than 18–24 months and it is accompanied by the integration of viral DNA into eukaryotic DNA in basal cells, may be associated with malignant and potentially malignant development [73]. This latter form of infection is recognized as the cause of CSCC. Clinically, HPV infects basal cells of the skin's epithelium and mucous membranes [73]. Because HPV can affect the site of epithelial cells, infections are found in the oral mucosa, esophagus, larynx, trachea, conjunctiva as well as the genitals and rectum [74]. This phenomenon explains the increased frequency of HPV-related OSCC [29].

Oral HPV infection can be acquired by oral-genital contact, by mouth-to-mouth contact, or possibly by autoinoculation and in infants by mother-to-child transmission [35]. The natural history of HPV infection in the oral cavity and oropharynx is not entirely clear although there are some characteristics similar to those described for the cervix of the uterus [75]. Histological similarities between the service vaginal and oropharyngeal regions, both coated with squamous epithelium or slightly keratin, and the capacity of the virus to perpetuate human oral keratinocytes in vitro, make it possible to transfer the concept of HPV induction oncogenicity occurring in gynecology to the oral cavity [76]. Although the way HPV is transmitted in the oral cavity is still not fully known, epidemiological data shows that detection of HPV (i.e. HPV 16) in chipped cells in the mouth increases the risk more than 14 times that of oropharyngeal cancer (tonsils and base of the tongue) and 3.8 times the risk of oral cancer [77, 78]. Syrjänen et al.'s findings suggest that the oral mucosa is a reservoir of infection, the virus can easily pass through the oral cavity and sometimes remain at riskier sites, such as tonsil kriptus similar to cervical squamosa cell connections [18, 64, 79]. The target of viral infection can also be at sites where basal keratinocytes do not differentiate [80]. The results of the meta-analysis Kreimer et al. detected confirmed the presence of HPV in the oral mucosa and showed only 4.5% (95% CI: 3.9–5.1) of the 4070 positive subjects for HPV and 3.5% (95% CI: 3.0–4.1) of the 4441 subjects had HPV carcinogenic mucosa and concluded the oral mucosa was a reservoir of infection [81]. Dayakar, Shipilova and Gupta's research shows more precisely that the reservoir is located in the gingiva pocket [82].

The oral cavity is a significant reservoir for HPV infection that may not be entirely independent of the cervical reservoir [35]. Because the high discordance of infections may reflect differences in the risk factors for or natural history of infection at the two sites, it may not be entirely appropriate to extrapolate the vast literature on cervical HPV natural history to oral HPV infection [35, 83].

3.4 HPV and oral potentially malignant disorders (OPMDs)

A large number of oral cancers are preceded by visible clinical changes that occur in the oral mucosa in the form of chronic white or red patches [84]. Some lesions and this condition carry malignant potential and are listed as premalignant [85]. WHO (2005) recommends that the term lesions and oral pre-malignant conditions be replaced with the term OPMDs. Based on these recommendations, oral leukoplakia (OL), oral erythroplakia (OE), oral proliferative verrucous leukoplakia (PVL), oral submucosal fibrosis, oral lichen planus (OLP) and actinic cheilitis have been classified as OPMD [86, 87].

A subgroup of HPVs, The HR-HPVs, can cause precancerous lesions [19]. Recent investigations of significant HPV detection rates are recorded in several OPMDs. Studies have reported the prevalence rate of HPV's relationship with OPMD ranges from 0–85% [88]. The most common OPMDs are OL, PVL, OE, and OLP [86]. OL, the most common disorder among OPMD and therefore the most studied in the literature, current evidence suggests that OL shows an increased risk of HPV infection with respect to clinically healthy mucosa, with a prevalence of about 20%, without significant differences in clinical presentation [89]. OE is a rare OPMD characterized by a large neoplastic risk [90]. Due to its very low frequency, references to viral infections are very rare in the literature. The latest data published by Syrjänen et al. reported that of the 11 OE tested for HPV, 54.5% were found to be HPV positive 16 [90]. OLP is also associated with viral infections, with the frequency of infections ranging from 27 to 65% [90]. Some authors hypothesize the influence of erosive OLP in increasing the risk of HPV infection, although this hypothesis has not been confirmed by subsequent research [91]. In the review Syrjänen et al. prevalence of HPV infection in OLP was 5.12%, with genotype 16 most commonly involved [29].

In the context of maligna's transformation from OPMD, the potential role of HPV promoters is still debated. Szarka et al. reported an increase in HPV prevalence in OPMD with increased malignant potential: 32.8%, 40.9% and 47.7% in OLP, OL and OSCC [92].

4. Dental calculus: novel promising biosource for HPV-induced oral cancer study

The oral cavity is a place where various microorganisms live. On the surface of teeth, supra or subgingival, the biofilm of these microorganisms with the additional contribution of saliva and gingival crevicular fluids (GCF) can calcify into dental calculus [93]. This process starts with the formation of plaque. A thin layer (film) of salivary protein will adhere to the surface of the tooth. It is then called the acquired enamel pellicle (AEP). AEP is the main barrier between the enamel and bacteria and food acids. The next layer is a colony of microorganisms with a bacterial density of more than 200 million bacterial cells per milligram. Plaque is bound by a matrix of bacterial extracellular polymeric substances (EPSs), in which desquamated cells, oral microorganisms, food debris, microscopic particles, and biomolecules such as DNA, RNA and protein can be trapped [93–95]. Calcium phosphate ions from saliva and GCF can also affect this process [49, 96].

Calcium phosphate is the most dominant mineral in dental calculus. The calcification process occurs periodically, beginning from the layer closest to the teeth, so each layer has a different morphology and stoichiometric composition. Hydroxyapatite (HAP) is the layer that sticks to the surface of teeth. The next layers, from inside to the outside, are layers of whitlockite (TCP-b), octocalcium phosphate (OCP), and brushite (B) [93]. Irregular tooth surfaces, pits and fissures are also predisposing factors for the accumulation of dental calculus [93, 94].

Dental calculus can be found in all human populations, in the past and at present, especially in groups of people with poor oral hygiene. Clinically it can be observed easily, and it accumulates around the neck of the teeth, causing chronic inflammation of the periodontal tissue. This condition causes the formation of periodontal pockets. This hallmark periodontitis is an ideal reservoir for HPV [82, 97].

The target cells of HPV are cells in the basal layer because they have a high proliferation capacity, so they can support the replication of the virus [70, 98]. In the periodontal pocket, the basal layer is exposed to the outside environment [97]. The junctional epithelium in this area has a high proliferative capacity [70, 82, 97]. Virions bind initially to the glycosaminoglycan (GAG) chains of the heparan sulphate proteoglycan (HSPG) of epithelial cells [4]. This protein is expressed more in the healing process in the periodontal pocket [97, 99].

GCF is a very specific oral cavity fluid that represents periodontal health [99]. In several studies, this fluid has been used as a biological source of detection for the presence of HPV [97, 100]. HPV DNA is detected in advanced cases of periodontitis, but not detected in patients with gingivitis [101, 102]. There is a tendency that it is detected more often in women [100]. Women's specific factors, such as decreased levels of sex hormones, may increase the risk of HPV infection in the periodontal pocket [103].

HPV has several characteristics including selecting basal cells as its target, being latent, and its virions being released into the external environment together with desquamated cells [104]. Desquamated cells from the entire mouth will be carried in saliva, some of which will be precipitated into dental calculus. Saliva only shows the state of the moment [105]. Meanwhile, the part that precipitates into dental calculus will last if it is has not been cleaned, so the dental calculus is able to store data longer and to be the evidence of the presence of HPV in the past. This is consistent with the latent nature of the HPV infection.

The involvement of HPV in cancer will greatly influence the treatment plan and prognosis, so detection of its involvement is very important [4, 106]. Various studies have been carried out to develop the examination designs. The method of examination, the molecular targets, and the biological sources used were considered in those studies [11, 106, 107].

Various methods have been developed, ranging from observation of tissue morphology to visualization of molecular markers. In microscopic observation, pathognomonic koilocytotic cells have been observed [108]. The HPV-infected cells show perinuclear halo, enlarged cell nucleus, increased ratio of nucleus and cytoplasm, dysplasia, and minimal keratinization [106, 108]. Observation of these morphological changes really depends on the operator's carefulness [106]. Various stains are used, from the most conventional – hematoxylin & eosin, Papanicolaou and immunohistochemical staining (IHC) [106, 109]. The protein used in IHC can HPV origin, for example E6 and E7 or p16 from host [110]. IHC staining method is simple but the results are less consistent [106]. HPV infection is latent, it takes a long time for the tissue to show pathognomonic signs [8].

The initial step in early detection of HPV-induced cancer is to confirm the presence of the virus [111]. HPV cannot be cultured in vitro [112]. Molecular analysis is developed to detect HPV even before tissue changes can be observed. The molecular targets include DNA, RNA, HPV proteins, and host antibodies [106]. The detection methods that can be used are nucleic acid-hybridization assays, signal amplification assays and nucleic-acid amplification [113]. Detection kits in various brands have been widely circulating in the market [112].

The biological source of samples also determines the detection of HPV. If the cancer is clinically visible, it is easier to determine the biological source. However, for early detection, the collection of the sample must be non-invasive, and the life cycle of HPV must be considered. This virus is epithelial tropism, infecting mainly cells in the basal layer. It is latent, and when it is mature, virions will exit the cell [4, 104].

Routine cytology examination for early detection of cervical cancer has become a health program in various countries [114, 115]. The oral cavity is very different from the cervix. The oral mucosa is very broad, with various anatomical landmarks more varied than those of the cervix. Several studies have used oral swabs, oral rinse, and saliva of non-oral cancer individuals [110, 116, 117]. These various biological sources represent only the condition of the oral cavity then, while HPV is latent [8]. No biological source has been acknowledged as the standard source in routine examinations of the oral cavity.

Dental calculus is formed from calcified plaque which can accumulate sub gingivally or supragingival [118]. During the maturation process, the dental calculus can trap organic material, for example cells with integrated viral genomes, DNA, RNA, proteins, molecules, and other biological data [93, 95]. This makes dental calculus a potential biological source for molecular examination of latent pathogens [95]. To our knowledge, for the first time, our study was able to detect the presence of latent HPV in the dental calculus of the periodontal pockets of patients with OSCC accompanied by chronic periodontitis. These results strongly suggest that dental calculus is a promising biological source for the detection of HPV in the oral cavity and can be used as a biomarker for early detection as shown in **Figure 1** [11].

DNA isolates from the dental calculus of OSCC patients were amplified with the universal primer MY09 /11. In visualization, 29% of the samples had a clear

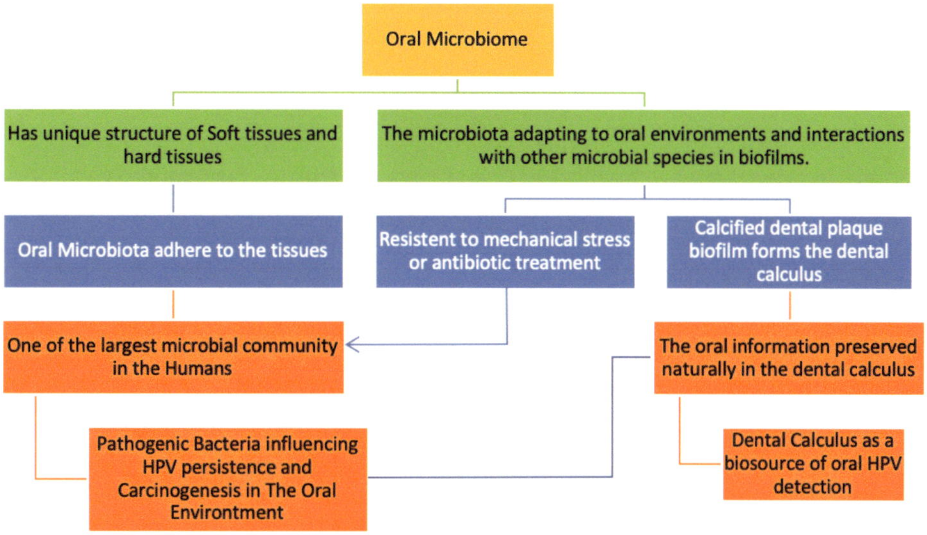

Figure 1.
Dental calculus as a potential biosource of HPV detection. This diagram shows the potential reasons why dental calculus will have an important role in the future of oral cancer study.

single band, at 450 bp. The Sanger method was performed to determine the DNA sequence, the sequence was compared with the data on GenBank using NCBI BLAST online on the website https://blast.ncbi.nlm.nih.gov [119]. HPV 58 was identified in 75% of the samples, while the rest was identified as unclassified HPV. Type 58 is included as high risk HPV and is the most common genotype found in cervical cancer after HPV 16 and 18 in East Asia and in Thailand [120, 121].

It is predicted that in 2035 there will be an increase in the global incidence of malignancies of the lips, oral cavity, and pharynx by about 62% [122]. It is also predicted that 95% of this malignancy is OSCC [123]. There have been only few studies about HPV genotype in the oral cavity, [124, 125]. so further studies need to be done to make sure this prediction will not come true. Interestingly, this study showed that the remaining positive samples were identified as unclassified papillomaviridae. Further research on unclassified HPV is still ongoing. This finding suggests the possibility of the presence of other papillomaviridae viruses that have not been identified.

The goal of any developing technology for HPV detection in clinical samples is to approach the gold standard for sensitivity and specificity while maximizing efficiency, simplicity, reproducibility, and transferability to the routine diagnostic laboratory. Our research is currently developing dental calculus as the standard of biological source for the detection of HPV in the oral cavity.

5. Conclusion

The oral cavity contains hundreds of different microorganisms that can associate to form biofilms. Biofilms are resistant to mechanical stress or antibiotic treatment. Oral cavity also has unique structure that cannot be found anywhere else in the human body. These conditions led oral cavity to become one of the largest microbial community in the humans. The oral plaque biofilm are calcified to dental calculus. During biomineral maturation process, several biological contents around the oral region should be trapped in dental calculus, including the exfoliated virus contained cells. Hence, dental calculus is a promising biosource of HPV and carcinogens molecules detection in the oral cavity.

Acknowledgements

All authors have made substantial contribution to this study and/or chapter, and all have reviewed the final paper prior to its submission. We thank to Faculty of Dentistry of Universitas Padjadjaran, and Faculty of Dentistry of Maranatha Christian University for the technical support during the research. This research received grant from Universitas Padjadjaran under Academic Leadership Grant #1427/UN6.3.1/LT/2020 and Maranatha Christian University.

Conflict of interest

The authors declare that there is no conflict of interest regarding the publication of this chapter.

Author details

Sunardhi Widyaputra[1]*, Natallia Pranata[2], Ignatius Setiawan[3] and Jamas Ari Anggraini[1]

1 Department of Oral Biology, Faculty of Dentistry, Universitas Padjadjaran, Bandung, Indonesia

2 Department of Oral Biology, Faculty of Dentistry, Maranatha Christian University, Bandung, Indonesia

3 Department of Dental Public Health, Faculty of Dentistry, Maranatha Christian University, Bandung, Indonesia

*Address all correspondence to: sunardhi.widyaputra@fkg.unpad.ac.id

References

[1] Candotto V, Laurintano D, Nardone M, Baggi L, Arcuri C, Gatto R, et al. HPV infection in the oral cavity: epidemiology, clinical manifestations and relationship with oral cancer. Oral & Implantology. 2017;10:209-220.

[2] Selby CC. An electron microscope study of the epidermis of mammalian skin in thin sections. J Biophys Biochem Cytol. 1955;1:429-444.

[3] Egawa N, Egawa K, Griffin H, Doorbar J. Human papillomaviruses; epithelial tropisms, and the development of neoplasia. Viruses. 2015;7:3863-3890.

[4] Medda A, Duca D, Chiocca S. Human papillomavirus and cellular pathways: hits and targets. Pathogens. Multidisciplinary Digital Publishing Institute; 2021;10:262.

[5] Human Reference clones – hpvcenter [Internet]. [cited 2021 Apr 13]. Available from: https://www.hpvcenter.se/human_reference_clones/

[6] Leemans CR, Braakhuis BJM, Brakenhoff RH. The molecular biology of head and neck cancer. Nature Reviews Cancer. 2011;11:9-22.

[7] Harden ME, Munger K. Human papillomavirus molecular biology. Mutat Res. 2017;772:3-12.

[8] IARC. Human papillomaviruses. in: biological agents. IARC Monographs. 2012;100B:255-315.

[9] Miranda-Galvis M, Loveless R, Kowalski LP, Teng Y. Impacts of environmental factors on head and neck cancer pathogenesis and progression. Cells. 2021;10:1-16.

[10] Brondani MA, Siqueira AB, Alves CMC. Exploring lay public and dental professional knowledge around HPV transmission via oral sex and oral cancer development. BMC Public Health. 2019;19:1-8.

[11] Pranata N, Maskoen AM, Sahiratmadja E, Widyaputra S. Dental Calculus as a Potential Biosource for Human papillomavirus detection in oral squamous cell carcinoma. Asian Pacific Journal of Cancer Prevention. West Asia Organization for Cancer Prevention (WAOCP), APOCP's West Asia Chapter; 2020;21:3093-3097.

[12] Sanjos S De, Brotons M, Angel M. The natural history of human papillomavirus infection. Best Practice & Research Clinical Obstetrics and Gynaecology. 2018;47:2-13.

[13] Bernard H. Review: The clinical importance of the nomenclature, evolution and taxonomy of human papillomaviruses. Journal of Clinical Virology. 2005;32:1-6.

[14] Wang CJ, Palefsky JM. Human Papillomavirus (HPV) Infections and the Importance of HPV Vaccination. Curr Epidemiol Rep. 2015;2:101-109.

[15] Ljubojević S, Lipozenčić J, Grgec DL, Prstačić R, Skerlev M, Mokos ZB. Human papilloma virus associated with genital infection. Collegium Antropologicum. 2008;32:989-997.

[16] Steben M, Duarte-franco E. Human papillomavirus infection : Epidemiology and pathophysiology. Gynecologic Oncology. 2007;107:2-5.

[17] Bernard HU, Burk RD, Chen Z, van Doorslaer K, Hausen H zur, de Villiers EM. Classification of papillomaviruses (PVs) based on 189 PV types and proposal of taxonomic amendments. Virology. Elsevier Inc.; 2010;401:70-9.

[18] Rautava J, Syrja S. Biology of Human papillomavirus infections in head and neck carcinogenesis. Head and Neck Pathology. 2012;6:S3-15.

[19] Rampias T, Sasaki C, Psyrri A. Molecular mechanisms of HPV induced carcinogenesis in head and neck. Oral Oncology. 2014;50:356-363.

[20] Frazer IH. Prevention of cervical cancer through papillomavirus vaccination. Nat Rev Immunol. 2004;4:46-55.

[21] Worsham MJ, Chen KM, Ghanem T, Stephen JK, Divine G. Epigenetic modulation of signal transduction pathways in HPV-associated HNSCC. Otolaryngol-Head Neck Surg. 2013;149:409-416.

[22] Hernández-López R, Lorincz AT, Torres-Ibarra L, Reuter C, Scibior-Bentkowska D, Warman R, et al. Methylation estimates the risk of precancer in HPV-infected women with discrepant results between cytology and HPV16/18 genotyping. Clin Epigenetics. 2019;11:1-12.

[23] Johannsen E, Lambert PF. Epigenetics of human papillomaviruses. Virology. 2013;445:205-212.

[24] Villiers E De. Cross-roads in the classification of papillomaviruses. Virology. 2013;445:2-10.

[25] De Villiers EM, Fauquet C, Broker TR, Bernard HU, Zur Hausen H. Classification of papillomaviruses. Virology. 2004;324:17-27.

[26] Willemsen A, Bravo IG. Origin and evolution of papillomavirus (onco) genes and genomes. Phil Trans R Soc B. 2019;374:1-10.

[27] Jackson R, Eade S, Zehbe I, Eade S, Zehbe I, Zehbe I. An epithelial organoid model with Langerhans cells for assessing virus-host interactions. Phil Trans R Soc B. 2019;374:1-11.

[28] Tommasino M. The human papillomavirus family and its role in carcinogenesis. Seminars in Cancer Biology. Elsevier Ltd; 2014;26:13-21.

[29] Rautava J, Syrjänen S. Human papillomavirus infections in the oral mucosa. J Am Dent Assoc. 2011;142:905-914.

[30] Quint KD, Genders RE, Koning MN de, Borgogna C, Gariglio M, Bavinck JNB, et al. Human Beta-papillomavirus infection and keratinocyte carcinomas. J Pathol. 2015;235:342-354.

[31] Wang H, Duffy AA, Broker TR, Chow LT. Robust production and passaging of infectious HPV in squamous epithelium of primary human keratinocytes. Genes & Development. 2009;23:181-194.

[32] Doorbar J. The papillomavirus life cycle. Journal of Clinical Virology. 2005;32S:7-15.

[33] Olivero C, Lanfredini S, Borgogna C, Gariglio M, Patel GK. HPV-induced field cancerisation : transformation of adult tissue stem cell into cancer stem cell. Frontiers in Microbiology. 2018;9:1-8.

[34] Bruni L, Albero G, Serrano B, Mena M, Gomez D, Munoz J, et al. Human papillomavirus and related diseases report. 2019.

[35] Fakhry C, Gypsyamber D, Sugar E, Weber K, Goshu E, Minkoff H, et al. Relationship between prevalent oral and cervical human papillomavirus infections in human immunodeficiency virus-positive and -negative women. Journal of Clinical Microbiology. 2006;44:4479-4485.

[36] Ang KK, Harris J, Wheeler R, Weber R, Rosenthal DI, Nguyen-Tan PF, et al. Human papillomavirus and survival of patients with oropharyngeal

cancer. The New England Journal of Medicine. 2010;363:24-35.

[37] Graham S V. The human papillomavirus replication cycle, and its links to cancer progression : a comprehensive review. Clinical Science. 2017;0:2201-2221.

[38] Bodily J, Laimins LA. Persistence of human papillomavirus infections: keys to malignant progression. Trends Microbiol. 2011;19:33-39

[39] Gollin SM. Epidemiology of HPV-associated oropharyngeal squamous cell carcinoma. In: Miller DL, Stack MS, editors. Human papillomavirus (HPV) -associated oropharyngeal cancer. Springer International Publishing; 2015. p. 2-3.

[40] Mclaughlin-drubin ME, Münger K. The human papillomavirus E7 oncoprotein. Virology. 2009;384:335-344.

[41] Moody CA, Laimins LA. Human papillomavirus oncoproteins : pathways to transformation. Nature Publishing Group. 2010;10:550-560.

[42] Leeman AD, Jenkins D, Marra E, Zummeren M Van, Pirog EC, Sandt MM Van De, et al. Grading immunohistochemical markers p16 INK4a and HPV E4 identifies productive and transforming lesions caused by low- and high-risk HPV within high-grade anal squamous intraepithelial lesions. British Journal of Dermatology. 2020;182:1026-1033.

[43] Deo PN, Deshmukh R. Oral microbiome: Unveiling The Fundamentals. Journal of Oral and Maxillofacial Pathology. 2019;23:122-128.

[44] Tuominen H, Rautava J. Oral microbiota and cancer development. Pathobiology. 2021;88:116-126.

[45] E.Blum H. The Human microbiome. Advances in Medical Sciences. 2017;6:414-420.

[46] Lin D, Kouzy R, Jaoude JA, Noticewala SS, Medrano AYD, Klopp AH, et al. Microbiome factors in HPV-driven carcinogenesis and cancers. PLOS Pathogens. 2020;16:1-8.

[47] Francesco De Seta, Giuseppina Campisciano, Nunzia Zanotta, Giuseppe Ricci, Manola Comar. The vaginal community state types microbiome-immune network as key factor for bacterial vaginosis and aerobic vaginitis. Frotiers in Microbiology. 2019;10:1-8.

[48] Maria Avila, David M. Ojcius, Özlem Yilmaz. The oral microbiota: living with a permanent guest. DNA and Cell Biology. 2009;28:405-411.

[49] Newman MG, Takei HH, Klokkevold PR, Carranza FA. Newman and Carranza's Clinical Periodontologi. 13th ed. Philadelphia: Elseiver; 2019.

[50] Zhang L, Liu Y, Zheng HJ, Zhang CP. The oral microbiota may have influence on oral cancer. Front Cell Infect Microbiol. Frontiers; 2020;9:1-11.

[51] Rafael Guerrero-Preston, James Robert White, Filipa Godoy-Vitorino, Arnold Rodríguez-Hilario, Kelvin Navarro, Herminio González, et al. High-resolution microbiome profiling uncovers Fusobacterium nucleatum, Lactobacillus Gasseri/Johnsonii, and Lactobacillus Vaginalis associated to oral and oropharyngeal cancer in saliva from HPV positive and HPV negative patients treated with surgery and chemo-radiation. Oncotarget. 2017; 8:110931-110948.

[52] Coussens LM, Werb Z. Inflammation and cancer. Nature. 2002;420:860-867.

[53] Loesche WJ, Grossman NS. Periodontal disease as a specific, albeit

chronic, infection: diagnosis and treatment. Clin Microbiol Rev. 2001;14:727-752.

[54] Burt B. Epidemiology of Periodontal Diseases. J Periodontol. 2005;76:1406-1419.

[55] Armitage GC. Periodontal diagnoses and classification of periodontal diseases. Periodontology 2000. 2004;34:9-21.

[56] Irfan M, Delgado RZR, Frias-Lopez J. The oral microbiome and cancer. Front Immunol. 2020;11:1-18.

[57] Groeger S, Domann E, Gonzales JR, Chakraborty T, Meyle J. B7-H1 and B7-DC receptors of oral squamous carcinoma cells are upregulated by Porphyromonas gingivalis. Immunobiology. 2011;216:1302-1310.

[58] Hoare A, Soto C, Rojas-Celis V, Bravo D. Chronic inflammation as a link between periodontitis and carcinogenesis. Mediators Inflamm. 2019;1-14.

[59] Kipanyula MJ, Seke Etet PF, Vecchio L, Farahna M, Nukenine EN, Nwabo Kamdje AH. Signaling pathways bridging microbial-triggered inflammation and cancer. Cellular Signalling. 2013;25:403-416.

[60] Li Y, Tan X, Zhao X, Xu Z, Dai W, Duan W, et al. Composition and function of oral microbiota between gingival squamous cell carcinoma and periodontitis. Oral Oncol. 2020;107:104710-104721.

[61] Giuliano AR, Nyitray AG, Kreimer AR, Campbell CMP, Goodman MT, Sudenga SL, et al. Differences in human papillomavirus related cancer incidence by gender and anatomic site of infection. Int J Cancer. 2016;136:2752-2760.

[62] Ljubojevic S, Skerlev M. HPV-associated diseases. Clin Dermatol. 2014;32:227-234

[63] Feller L, Khammissa RAG, Wood NH, Lemmer J. Epithelial maturation and molecular biology of oral HPV. 2009;9:1-9.

[64] Syrjänen S. HPV infections and tonsillar carcinoma. J Clin Pathol. 2004;57:449-455.

[65] Rodríguez AC, Schiffman M, Herrero R, Wacholder S, Hildesheim A, Castle PE, et al. Rapid clearance of human papillomavirus and implications for clinical focus on persistent infections. J Natl Cancer Inst. 2008;100:513-517.

[66] Day PM, Schelhaas M. Concepts of papillomavirus entry into host cells. Curr Opin Virol. 2014;February:24-31.

[67] Dell G, Wilkinson KW, Tranter R, Parish J, Brady RL, Gaston K. Comparison of the structure and DNA-binding properties of the E2 proteins from an oncogenic and a non-oncogenic human papillomavirus. J Mol Biol. 2003;334:979-991.

[68] Doorslaer K Van. Evolution of the papillomaviridae. Virology. Elsevier; 2013;445:11-20.

[69] Juckett G, Hartman-Adams H. Human papillomavirus: Clinical manifestations and prevention. American Family Physician. 2010;82:1209-1214.

[70] Syrjänen S. Oral manifestations of human papillomavirus infections. European Journal of Oral Sciences. 2018;126:49-66.

[71] Pringle GA. The role of human papillomavirus in oral disease. Dent Clin North Am. 2014;58:385-399.

[72] Betz SJ. HPV-related papillary lesions of the oral mucosa: A review. Head Neck Pathol. 2019;13:80-90.

[73] Trottier H, Burchell AN. Epidemiology of mucosal human

papillomavirus infection and associated diseases. Public Health Genomics. 2009;12:291-307.

[74] Grce M, Mravak-stipeti M. Human papillomavirus – associated diseases. Clinics in Dermatology. 2014;32:253-258.

[75] D'Souza G, Fakhry C, Sugar EA, Seaberg EC, Weber K, Minkoff HL, et al. Six-month natural history of oral versus cervical human papillomavirus infection. International Journal of Cancer. 2007;121:143-150.

[76] Sanders AE, Slade GD, Patton LL. National prevalence of oral HPV infection and related risk factors in the US adult population reply. Oral Diseases. 2013;19:106.

[77] D'Souza G, Kreimer AR, Viscidi R, Pawlita M, Fakhry C, Koch WM, et al. Case–control study of human papillomavirus and oropharyngeal cancer. New England Journal of Medicine. 2007;356:1944-1956.

[78] Chaturvedi AK, Engels EA, Pfeiffer RM, Hernandez BY, Xiao W, Kim E, et al. Human papillomavirus and rising oropharyngeal cancer incidence in the United States. Journal of Clinical Oncology. 2011;29:4294-4301.

[79] Campisi G, Giovannelli L. Controversies surrounding human papilloma virus infection, head & neck vs oral cancer, implications for prophylaxis and treatment. Head & neck oncology. 2009;1:8.

[80] Spoden G, Kuhling L, Cordes N, Frenzel B, Sapp M, Boller K, et al. Human papillomavirus types 16, 18, and 31 share similar endocytic requirements for entry. Journal of Virology. 2013;87:7765-7773.

[81] Kreimer AR, Bhatia RK, Messeguer AL, González P, Herrero R, Giuliano AR. Oral human papillomavirus in healthy individuals: A systematic review of the literature. Sexually Transmitted Diseases. 2010;37:386-391.

[82] Dayakar M, Shipilova A, Gupta D. Periodontal pocket as a potential reservoir of high risk human papilloma virus: A pilot study. Journal of Indian Society of Periodontology. 2016;20:136-140.

[83] Herrero R, Castellsagué X, Pawlita M, Lissowska J, Kee F, Balaram P, et al. Human papillomavirus and oral cancer: The international agency for research on cancer multicenter study. Journal of the National Cancer Institute. 2003;95:1772-1783.

[84] Hosni ES, Salum FG, Cherubini K, Yurgel LS, Figueiredo MAZ. Oral erythroplakia and speckled leukoplakia: retrospective analysis of 13 cases. Brazilian Journal of Otorhinolaryngology. 2009;75:295-299.

[85] Watanabe N, Ohkubo T, Shimizu M, Tanaka T. Preneoplasia and carcinogenesis of the oral cavity. Oncol Discov. 2015;3:1-12.

[86] Dionne KR, Warnakulasuriya S, Zain RB, Cheong SC. Potentially malignant disorders of the oral cavity: Current practice and future directions in the clinic and laboratory. International Journal of Cancer. 2015;136:503-515.

[87] Warnakulasuriya S, Johnson NW, Waal I Van Der. Nomenclature and classification of potentially malignant disorders of the oral mucosa. J Oral Pathol Med. 2007;36:575-580.

[88] Bouda M, Gorgoulis VG, Kastrinakis NG, Giannoudis A, Tsoli E, Danassi-Afentaki D, et al. "High risk" HPV types are frequently detected in potentially malignant and malignant oral lesions, but not in normal oral mucosa. Modern Pathology. 2000;13:644-653.

[89] Termine N, Giovannelli L, Rodolico V, Matranga D, Pannone G, Campisi G. Biopsy vs. brushing: Comparison of two sampling methods for the detection of HPV-DNA in squamous cell carcinoma of the oral cavity. Oral Oncol. 2012;48:870-875.

[90] Syrjänen S, Lodi G, Bultzingslowen I von, Aliko A, Arduino P, Campisi G, et al. Human papillomaviruses in oral carcinoma and oral potentially malignant disorders : a systematic review. Oral Diseases. 2011;17:58-72.

[91] Shang Q, Peng J, Zhou Y, Chen Q, Xu H. Association of human papillomavirus with oral lichen planus and oral leukoplakia: A meta-analysis. J Evid Based Dent Pract. 2020;20:1-13.

[92] Szarka K, Tar I, Fehér E, Gáll T, Kis A, Tóth ED, et al. Progressive increase of human papillomavirus carriage rates in potentially malignant and malignant oral disorders with increasing malignant potential. Oral Microbiol Immunol. 2009;24:314-318.

[93] Warinner C, Speller C, Collins MJ. A new era in palaeomicrobiology: prospects for ancient dental calculus as a long-term record of the human oral microbiome. Philosophical Transactions of the Royal Society B: Biological Sciences. 2014;370:1-11.

[94] Brundin M, Figdor D, Sundqvist G, Sjögren U. DNA binding to hydroxyapatite: A potential mechanism for preservation of microbial DNA. Journal of Endodontics. 2013;39:211-216.

[95] Metcalf JL, Ursell LK, Knight R. Ancient human oral plaque preserves a wealth of biological data. Nat Genet. 2014;46:321-323.

[96] Pranata N. Dental calculus as the unique calcified oral ecosystem a review article. Oceana Biomedicina Journal. 2019;2:52-65.

[97] Hormia M, Willberg J, Ruokonen H, Syrjänen S. Marginal periodontium as a potential reservoir of human papillomavirus in oral mucosa. Journal of periodontology. 2005;76:358-363.

[98] Pullos AN, Castilho RM, Squarize CH. HPV infection of the head and neck region and its stem cells. Journal of dental research. 2015;94:1532-1543.

[99] Khurshid Z, Mali M, Naseem M, Najeeb S, Zafar MS. Human Gingival Crevicular Fluids (GCF) Proteomics: An Overview. Dent J. 2017;5:1-8.

[100] Shigeishi H, Murodumi H, Ohta K, Sugiyama M. Detection of HPV16 E6 DNA in periodontal pockets of middle-aged and older people. Oral Science International. 2021;18:50-55.

[101] Parra B, Slots J. Detection of human viruses in periodontal pockets using polymerase chain reaction. Oral Microbiology and Immunology. 1996;11:289-293.

[102] Tezal M, Sullivan Nasca M, Stoler DL, Melendy T, Hyland A, Smaldino PJ, et al. Chronic periodontitis–human papillomavirus synergy in base of tongue cancers. Arch Otolaryngol Head Neck Surg. 2009;135:391.

[103] Marks MA, Gravitt PE, Burk RD, Studentsov Y, Farzadegan H, Klein SL. Progesterone and 17β-estradiol enhance regulatory responses to human papillomavirus type 16 Virus-like particles in peripheral blood mononuclear cells from healthy women. Clin Vaccine Immunol. 2010;17:609-617.

[104] Kajitani N, Satsuka A, Kawate A, Sakai H. Productive lifecycle of human papillomaviruses that depends upon squamous epithelial differentiation. Front Microbiol. 2012;3:1-12.

[105] Jasim H, Olausson P, Hedenberg-Magnusson B, Ernberg M,

Ghafouri B. The proteomic profile of whole and glandular saliva in healthy pain-free subjects. Sci Rep. 2016;6:1-10.

[106] Westra WH. Detection of human papillomavirus in clinical samples. Otolaryngologic Clinics of North America. 2012;45:765-777.

[107] Sastre-Garau X, Harlé A. Pathology of HPV-associated head and neck carcinomas: recent data and perspectives for the development of specific tumor markers. Front Oncol. 2020;10:528957.

[108] Krawczyk E, Suprynowicz FA, Liu X, Dai Y, Hartmann DP, Hanover J, et al. Koilocytosis. Am J Pathol. 2008;173:682-688.

[109] Fletcher S. Histopathology of papilloma virus infection of the cervix uteri: the history, taxonomy, nomenclature and reporting of koilocytic dysplasias. J Clin Pathol. 1983;36:616-624.

[110] Wimardhani YS, Sasanti H, Wardhany II, Sarsito AS, Pradono SA, Subita GP, et al. Saliva-based screening of high-risk human papillomavirus strains: detection in female Indonesian and Thai dental students. Asian Pacific Journal of Cancer Prevention. 2015;16:5525-5529.

[111] Bruhn LV, Andersen SJ, Hariri J. HPV-testing versus HPV-cytology co-testing to predict the outcome after conization. Acta Obstetricia et Gynecologica Scandinavica. 2018;97:758-765.

[112] Torres M, Fraile L, Echevarria J, Hernandez Novoa B, Ortiz M. Human papillomavirus (HPV) genotyping: Automation and application in routine laboratory testing. Open Virol J. 2012;6:144-150.

[113] Abreu AL, Souza RP, Gimenes F, Consolaro ME. A review of methods for detect human papillomavirus infection. Virology journal. 2012;9:262-271.

[114] Camacho R, Sepúlveda C, Neves D, Piñeros M, Villanueva M, Dangou J-M, et al. Cancer control capacity in 50 low- and middle-income countries. Glob Public Health. 2015;10:1017-1031.

[115] Anwar SL, Tampubolon G, Van Hemelrijck M, Hutajulu SH, Watkins J, Wulaningsih W. Determinants of cancer screening awareness and participation among Indonesian women. BMC Cancer. 2018;18:1-11.

[116] Goot-Heah K, Kwai-Lin T, Froemming GRA, Abraham MT, Rosdy NMMNM, Zain RB. Human papilloma virus 18 detection in oral squamous cell carcinoma and potentially malignant lesions using saliva samples. Asian Pacific Journal of Cancer Prevention. 2012;13:6109-6113.

[117] Shigeishi H, Sugiyama M. Risk factors for oral human papillomavirus infection in healthy individuals: A systematic review and meta-analysis. Journal of Clinical Medicine Research. 2016;8:721-729.

[118] Weyrich LS, Dobney K, Cooper A. Ancient DNA analysis of dental calculus. Journal of Human Evolution. 2015;79:119-124.

[119] Johnson M, Zaretskaya I, Raytselis Y, Merezhuk Y, McGinnis S, Madden TL. NCBI BLAST: a better web interface. Nucleic Acids Res. 2008;36:W5–W9.

[120] Panigoro R, Susanto H, Novel SS, Hartini S, Sahiratmadja E. HPV genotyping linear assay test comparison in cervical cancer patients: implications for HPV prevalence and molecular epidemiology in a limited-resource area in Bandung, Indonesia. Asian Pacific Journal of Cancer Prevention. 2013;14:5843-5847.

[121] Khunamornpong S, Settakorn J, Sukpan K, Suprasert P, Srisomboon J, Intaraphet S, et al. Genotyping for human papillomavirus (HPV) 16/18/52/58 has a higher performance than HPV16/18 genotyping in triaging women with positive high-risk HPV test in Northern Thailand. PLOS ONE. 2016;11:1-15.

[122] Ferlay J, Soerjomataram I, Dikshit R, Eser S, Mathers C, Rebelo M, et al. Cancer incidence and mortality worldwide: Sources, methods and major patterns in GLOBOCAN 2012: Globocan 2012. International Journal of Cancer. 2015;136:359-386.

[123] Shield KD, Ferlay J, Jemal A, Sankaranarayanan R, Chaturvedi AK, Bray F, et al. The global incidence of lip, oral cavity, and pharyngeal cancers by subsite in 2012. CA: A Cancer Journal for Clinicians. 2017;67:51-64.

[124] Bottalico D, Chen Z, Dunne A, Ostoloza J, McKinney S, Sun C, et al. The oral cavity contains abundant known and novel human papillomaviruses from the Betapapillomavirus and Gammapapillomavirus genera. The Journal of Infectious Diseases. 2011;204:787-792.

[125] Martin E, Dang J, Bzhalava D, Stern J, Edelstein ZR, Koutsky LA, et al. Characterization of three novel human papillomavirus types isolated from oral rinse samples of healthy individuals. J Clin Virol. 2014;59:30-37.

Section 3

Prevention and Control

Chapter 5

Preventing Human Papilloma Virus through Community Education and Vaccination

Celeste Mulry Baldwin and Lisa Rinke

Abstract

Human Papilloma Virus (HPV) affects many members of the community. To better educate the community in a participatory manner, engaging those outside of the health care arena is necessary. To prevent the spread of the disease in the United States, reaching the parents of children at the vulnerable age of 9–11 years of age is critical. The barriers to education of parents and children around the spread of a sexually transmitted disease are vast and difficult to overcome. However, the use of proven vaccinations give healthcare providers and community advocates the main tool for prevention of the spread of the disease. It is often taboo to discuss anything related to sexual promiscuity or sexual activity in the United States in the public schools. The biggest myth includes the fear parents and grandparents have is that if HPV is talked about, then the child may become sexually active sooner. This myth needs to be challenged with science and reality including taking on the those vehemently opposed to vaccines, known as "Anti-Vaxers" that obstruct vaccine education. The strategies utilized in public health outreach to the community should be reviewed and uniquely developed for each diverse community to overcome the challenges in the prevention of HPV.

Keywords: Human Papilloma Virus, HPV Vaccines, Preventable Cancers, Vaccine Hesitancy, Community Education, HPV Vaccine Rates in the United States

1. Introduction

Human Papilloma Virus (HPV) is a sexually transmitted disease that is found in multiple organs in both male and female patients. The role of the provider in this case is extremely vital in reducing the spread of the disease and encouraging vaccines for prevention of cancers. HPV is the one virus that has over 200 variants, which has an effective vaccine regimen available and provides coverage to eliminate the risk for fatal cancers [1]. Thus, it would seem to be an obvious step for children ages 9–11 years of age and those 11–45 years of age to receive the vaccine, yet that is not the case [2]. Less than 30% of children actually receive the vaccine and often, the second dose is avoided.

This vaccine hesitancy is a global issue in that some children live in poverty and do not have access to this preventable cancer vaccine and in addition, those children with high socio-economic statues refusing to be vaccinated at the advice of their parents. With regard to those 11–45 years of age, often this age group has not been fully educated about the concern over HPV infection and have concerns that they may get the disease.

Lastly, parental and grandparent vaccine hesitancy is due in part to lack of knowledge and concerns that the child may become promiscuous when vaccinated. Dispelling all of the myths surrounding HPV and the vaccine makes it difficult at best for providers to do due diligence in educating and preventing HPV. Which is quite distressing when over 13,00 cases of cervical cancers are diagnosed yearly in the United States (U.S.) and thousands of fatal cancers could be prevented [3].

This chapter outlines and provides the background including the incidence, prevalence, etiology, pathology, and health promotion measures of HPV. To appreciate HPV an understanding of regular screening and clinical practice guidelines are presented. The importance of health promotion and prevention is outlined. The goal of this chapter is to review the management and care to prevent HPV and subsequent complications, as well as present HPV vaccine rates, HPV vaccine hesitancy, and strategies to provide prevention at the community level.

1.1 Prevalence and incidence of HPV

As the fourth most common cancer, cervical cancer (CC) is a global health issue [4]. It is estimated that 75% of women will contract a HPV infection during their lifetime [5]. The annual incidence rate in the United States is 14 million [6]. A notable variability in the incidence rates of HPV exist worldwide. So, to are the disparities in detection and death of HPV. Tanzania reports 10,000 cases with 7000 death per year [4]. In Korean women, CC ranks as the seventh most common cancer [7]. As a result, the pathological manifestations of HPV may occur in the genital region and oral cavity [5]. Uterine cervical cancer incidence is approximately 600,000 cases per year. In oral pathogenesis, HPV 16 is likely to the primary cause accounting for 90% of malignant neoplasms [5].

According to the Centers for Disease Control (CDC), 40 out of the over 200 types of HPV can infect the genital region [8]. Despite being self-limited, asymptomatic, or unrecognized, sexual activity persons are likely to have become infected at least once. The most common types of oncogenic HPV, specifically 16 and 18, are responsible for the development of cervical, vulvar, vaginal, penile, anal, and oral pharyngeal cancer. Lower risk HPV type 6 and 11 are associated with respiratory papillomatosis and genital warts [8].

The prevalence of oral HPV in the United States between 2011 and 2014 was 7.3% in adults aged 18–69. During the same time frame, non-Hispanics saw a 2.9% rate and non- Hispanic black adults was 9.7% in comparison to 7.3% in non-Hispanic whites and 7% in Hispanic adults. Low prevalence rates occurred among non- Hispanic Asian women with no significance differences noted in non-Hispanic white, non-Hispanic black and Hispanic women. Overall, oral HPV was highest in men within each race and Hispanic group [9].

1.2 Most vulnerable populations that acquire HPV

According to the World Health Organization, greater than 85% of the 300,000 reported deaths from CC occur in countries with low to middle income. These rates are largely due to vaccination programs and screening practice in countries with higher income earnings [10]. Efforts to reach vulnerable populations are now distempered by the ongoing global pandemic due to the novel coronavirus (COVID-19), delaying and disrupting routine immunizations impinging accessibility, furthering inequalities of health care potentiating healthcare consequences globally [11].

2. The historical perspective of HPV

Nearly 528,000 women are diagnosed with cervical cancer each year with nearly half of them deceased [12]. The authors suggest that nearly 80% of the cases are found in third world countries are lacking the resources to battle this number of deaths. The evolution of (HPV) in the world is multifactorial leaving women in vulnerable populations more likely to contract one of the over 200 types most often through sexual transmission. The higher risk for women is due in part to the factors that lead to spread of HPV infection. Namely, early age at marriage, intercourse, pregnancy, and use of hormonal contraceptives [12]. Nearly 75% of adults that are sexually active have the disease without symptoms.

2.1 The evolution of HPV and types

There are over 200 types of HPV with 14 strains considered to be associated with cervical cancer [13]. Nearly 80 million people in the United States have been infected with most clearing the infection without incident [14]. In addition, these authors suggest that there has been a surge in oropharyngeal cancers related to HPV infection with the more notorious strains as the culprit [14].

2.2 Sites of origin of HPV

HPV is drawn to squamous epithelial cells and these are often found on mucosa such as skin and moist areas. HPV is most commonly found in the female cervix, however other sites of infection include those organs with similar tissue qualities such as the oropharynx, tonsillar tissue, soft palate, penis, and anus as examples. HPV tends to also live in the vagina, nose, nasopharynx, trachea, bronchi, and inner eyelid [15]. Frequently, HPV lives on the skin in the form of warts, however these growths can appear inside the organs described. Prevention of spread of anogenital warts is critical to decreasing the progression of cancer in males and females alike [16].

2.3 The diagnosis of HPV

The diagnosis of HPV is completed by performing a Papanicolaou (Pap) screening to identify infected cervical tissue [17]. This screening method first utilized in 1950's remains a gold standard for diagnosis. Cervical cancer remains the 4th most common cause of cancer in women globally [18]. The American Cancer Society (ACS) recommends that cervical cancer screening should begin at age 25 for women with an HPV test every five years using the U.S. Food and Drug Administration (FDA) tests only [15]. Those with higher risks such as immunocompromise include patients with HIV infection, organ transplant, or long term use of steroids [15]. If the patient has had a total hysterectomy with cervix removal and are cancer free are exempt from this testing.

2.4 Risks for preventable cancers

Cervical cancer evolves in four major steps, which include infection, persistence, progression, and invasion [18]. When the patient presents to clinic with oropharyngeal growths on the tongue or soft palate, a biopsy of the site should be performed and a follow up appointment should be scheduled once the diagnosis is confirmed. Most of the 230 genotypes of HPV cause no harm and resolve asymptomatically without the patient noticing with 40 genotypes known to be high risk [19]. Genital warts are tumors found caused by HPV, are the most common sexually transmitted disease, and generally are benign [19]. Risk factors for genital warts include: number of partners, barrier contraception use, young age at first encounter, circumcision, and male sexual behavior [19]. This high rate of transmission results in infection of multiple partners including females.

However, the clinician should be aware that correlating lymph node enlargement may require further biopsy to assure that squamous cell carcinoma is not in the tissue or lymph nodes. While most head and neck cancers are caused by squamous cell carcinoma and found historically in smoker, drinker, males >50 years of age, more recently it has been found in women in the oropharynx. This is occurring more often in the last decade as teens and young women engage in oral sex as a means to prevent pregnancy. In addition, males having sex with males are in a high risk category for this type of cancer due to multiple partners, as well as high risk for genital warts and anogenital cancer [19]. Recently, an anal Pap smear was created to help diagnose HPV in males having sex with multiple male partners. Recently, HPV is a culprit linked to urothelial bladder cancer as well [20].

3. Current treatments for HPV

A quadrivalent vaccine for HPV was first recommended by a sub-committee of the (CDC) in the United States known as the Advisory Committee on Immunization Practices (ACIP) in 2006 [21]. In 2009, a bivalent was available and in 2015, non-valent HPV vaccine was created and is the mainstay in HPV vaccination today. To date, the vaccine rates among girls ages 13–17 years of age remains quite low at nearly 42%, while boys in the same age group are worse at a rate of 28% [21]. Pediatricians and mid-level providers spend an inordinate amount of time working to educate families regarding this cancer prevention vaccine, yet compliance continues to be dismal. Adults should be vaccinated up until 45 years of age.

3.1 The target age group

The WHO Director in 2018, committed to eliminating cervical cancer with a significant goal of a 90% immunization rate in girls 15 years of age by 2030 [10]. Additionally, the Healthy People 2025 national goals in the U.S. continue to advocate for improved vaccine completion numbers. Approximately 70% of the global target population includes adolescent girls, ages 9–14, living in geographic regions without an immunization program for HPV prevention [21]. Adults less than 45 years of age are encouraged to take the vaccine.

3.2 Vaccine hesitancy

According to the WHO, if 70% vaccination coverage is achieved in low and middle income countries, approximate 4 million deaths could be prevented [10]. However, despite national recommendations, vaccine hesitancy often ensues [21]. In 2010 an estimated 14% of teenage girls in the USA completed and received all 3 doses, noting parental hesitancy as the primary reason for lack of follow through. One concern being the public policy mandate resulting in suspicion on the part of the parents. Parental opposition stems primarily from compulsory vaccination of their children citing trust and safety for the reluctance to pursue or complete the protocol. Several states in the U.S. require the HPV series to attend school, however, religious exemptions abound and this has not significantly increased the vaccination rate [22].

Knowledge served as a basis for hesitancy to vaccinate. However, parents with the higher levels of education tend to research the topic and decided against vaccination. Those with lower education levels tended to base decisions to vaccinate due to provide recommendation or encouragement opposed pursing knowledge or information regarding disease prevention with vaccination adherence [22]. Patient navigators to increase the vaccination rates and found that white patients are less likely to initiate the HPV vaccine than other ethnicities, however once initiated they were more likely to finish the series [22]. Rural parents were much less likely to encourage HPV vaccines as compared to their urban counterparts [13]. Women in the U.S. in general are basically poorly informed about HPV overall and found therefore, that provider education should target Non-Hispanic Blacks, lower level educated women, and those younger than 65 years of age. Beliefs about the efficacy of the vaccine to prevent cervical cancer remain a barrier to increased vaccine rates overall [22].

Parental attitudes toward vaccination of an STI factors into the decision-making process regarding vaccination prior to FDA approval. Several studies conducted demonstrated favorable attitudes in the USA and UK and accepting vaccination of their children. Specifically noting a mother's sexual values were secondary compared to overall vaccination attitude. In addition, social aversion to vaccination was not seen across various religions groups [23].

4. Community outreach

Cancer screening efforts are an ongoing effort to take the screening tools out to the community [3]. Educational outreach to vulnerable communities is an incredibly important method of reaching underserved groups. Often, vulnerable and underserved people are fearful of government institutions such as schools, social security, hospitals, and the police. The marginalized people in society have frequently been unsuccessful in navigating the system to obtain access to critical resources. In the case of Immigrants, the concern surrounds deportation or criminal charges. To overcome these barriers to educating and serving the public, healthcare providers are placed in the position of being more creative in how outreach is managed.

4.1 American Cancer Society (ACS) efforts

The American Cancer Society (ACS) has for decades provided funding, outreach, and resources to all patients in the U.S., as well as their regions and individual chapters. In the last decade, ACS has worked specifically to increase the knowledge base of parents, grandparents, and youth regarding the importance of cancer prevention, specifically for HPV. U.S. national immunization coalitions have devoted large amounts of time, effort, and funding to provide outreach for the public in an effort to prevent HPV. In 2014, a documentary about HPV and cervical cancer was produced in Hollywood called "Someone You Love: The HPV Epidemic." This documentary was shared at a conference in 2016 in Indianapolis, Indiana in the U.S. for a national meeting of all U.S. immunization coalitions. Soon, it spread throughout the U.S. as a tool for HPV prevention for youth and parents. It's real life powerful true stories of women that suffered and some died from cervical cancer caused by HPV. Other efforts in Maui, Hawai'i include having young cancer survivors assist in Relay for Life and ACS outreach events to speak candidly to youth about what HPV is and how disenchanting cancer treatment is along with the burden of fearing that the cancer may return.

Once the youth are aware of what the road for a cancer patient is like, they may not realize that there is one cancer that is preventable, and that is by vaccination against HPV.

5. Conclusion

Human Papilloma Virus (HPV) is the most common sexually transmitted disease that is found in in both male and female patients. The role of the provider in this case is extremely vital in reducing the spread of the disease and encouraging vaccines for prevention of cancers. HPV is the one virus that has over 200 variants, which has an effective vaccine regimen available and provides coverage to eliminate the risk for fatal cancers [1]. Thus, it would seem to be an obvious step for children ages 9–11 years of age and those 11–45 years of age to receive the vaccine, yet that is not the case [2]. Less than 30% of children actually receive the vaccine and often, the second dose is avoided.

Strategic elements to assist in global vaccination efforts include financial investment on a global level, enhancement of supply, single dose schedules, and effective social marketing [24]. Use of social media platforms to increase awareness of the notion that a vaccine preventable cancer such as cervical cancer may be the wave of the future. Without global concerted efforts to increase the vaccination rate to achieve herd immunity, the fight against HPV infection and the subsequent needless suffering and death will continue to occur.

Conflict of interest

The authors declare no conflict of interest.

Author details

Celeste Mulry Baldwin* and Lisa Rinke
DNP Online Graduate Program, Young School of Nursing, Regis College, Weston, MA, USA

*Address all correspondence to: celeste.baldwin@regiscollege.edu

References

[1] Senkomago V, Henley SJ, Thomas CC, Mix JM, Markowitz LE, Saraiya M. Human Papillomavirus–Attributable Cancers — United States, 2012-2016. MMWR Morb Mortal Wkly Rep 2019;68:724-728. DOI: http://dx.doi.org/10.15585/mmwr.mm6833a 3external icon.

[2] Meites E, Szilagyi PG, Chesson HW, Unger ER, Romero JR, Markowitz LE. Human Papillomavirus Vaccination for Adults: Updated Recommendations of the Advisory Committee on Immunization Practices. MMWR Morb Mortal Wkly Rep. 2019 Aug 16;68(32):698-702. doi: 10.15585/mmwr.mm6832a3. PMID: 31415491; PMCID: PMC6818701.

[3] Zhang, B.S. & Batur, P. (2019). Human papilloma virus in 2019: An update on cervical cancer and prevention and screening guidelines. Cleveland Clinic Journal of Medicine Volume 86, 3). MARCH 2019.

[4] Cooper EC, Maher JA, Naaseh A,et al. Implementation of human papillomavirus videoeducation for women participating in mass cervical cancer screening in Tanzania. Am J Obstet Gynecol. 2021;224:105.e1-9.

[5] Fiorillo L, Cervino G, Surace G, De Stefano R, Laino L, D'Amico C, Fiorillo MT, Meto A, Herford AS, Arzukanyan AV, Spagnuolo G, Cicciù M. Human Papilloma Virus: Current Knowledge and Focus on Oral Health. Biomed Res Int. 2021 Feb 1;2021:6631757. doi: 10.1155/2021/6631757. PMID: 33623784; PMCID: PMC7875628.

[6] Fueta, P. & Chido-Amajuoyi, O. Prevalence of HPV infection in the United States: A Comparison of HPV Infection Trends Pre and Post-HPV Vaccine Implementation. Pediatrics July 2020, 146 (1 MeetingAbstract) 571; DOI: https://doi.org/10.1542/peds.146.1_MeetingAbstract.571

[7] Kim, S.Y., Seo, J. W., & Ryu, E. (2021). Korean college students' attitudes and health behaviour regarding human papillomavirus vaccination. Volume 28, Issue 1, P. 57-62, February 01, 2021. Published: August 20, 2020DOI:https://doi.org/10.1016/j.colegn.2020.04.009

[8] Centers for Disease Control. Human papilloma virus (HPV) Fact Sheet https://www.cdc.gov/hpv/index.html. Accessed 04.20.21.

[9] McQuillan, G., Kruszon-Moran, D., Markowitz, L., Unger, & Paulose-Ram, R. Ph.D. National Health and Nutrition Examination Survey (NHANES) 2011-2014.

[10] World Health OrganizationWorld Health Organization. GLOBOCAN 2012 cancer incidence and mortality worldwide. Lyon (France): International Agency for Research on Cancer; 2016. [Google Scholar]. https://www.who.int/news-room/fact-sheets/detail/human-papillomavirus-(hpv)-and-cervical-cancer accessed 04.22.21.

[11] Toh ZQ, Russell FM, Garland SM, Mulholland EK, Patton G, Licciardi PV. Human Papillomavirus Vaccination After COVID-19. JNCI Cancer Spectr. 2021 Mar 2;5(2):pkab011. doi:

[12] Degarege A, Krupp K, Fennie K, Li T, Stephens DP, Marlow LAV, Srinivas V, Arun A, Madhivanan P. Urban-Rural Inequities in the Parental Attitudes and Beliefs Towards Human Papillomavirus Infection, Cervical Cancer, and Human Papillomavirus Vaccine in Mysore, India. J Pediatr Adolesc Gynecol. 2018 Oct;31(5):494-502. doi: 10.1016/j.jpag.2018.03.008. Epub 2018 Mar 26. PMID: 29596907; PMCID: PMC6119521.

[13] Chrysostomou, A. C., & Kostrikis, L. G. (2020). Methodologies of Primary HPV Testing Currently Applied for Cervical Cancer Screening. *Life (Basel, Switzerland)*, *10*(11), 290. https://doi.org/10.3390/life10110290

[14] Boakye, E., Tobo, B. B., Rojek, R., Mohammed, K.A., Geneus, C.J., & Osazuwa-Peters, N. (2017) Approaching a decade since HPV vaccine licensure: Racial and gender disparities in knowledge and awareness of HPV and HPV vaccine, Human Vaccines & Immunotherapeutics, 13:11, 2713-2722, DOI: 10.1080/21645515.2017.1363133

[15] American Cancer Society. (2021). https://www.cancer.org/cancer/cancer-causes/infectious-agents/hpv/hpv-and-hpv-testing.html.

[16] Skoulakis A, Fountas S, Mantzana-Peteinelli M, Pantelidi K, Petinaki E. Prevalence of human papillomavirus and subtype distribution in male partners of women with cervical intraepithelial neoplasia (CIN): a systematic review. BMC Infect Dis. 2019 Feb 26;19(1):192. doi: 10.1186/s12879-019-3805-x. PMID: 30808285; PMCID: PMC6390310.

[17] Hirth, J. (2019) Disparities in HPV vaccination rates and HPV prevalence in the United States: a review of the literature, Human Vaccines & Immunotherapeutics, 15:1, 146-155, DOI: 10.1080/21645515.2018.1512453

[18] Yamaguchi, Sekine, Hanley, Kudo, Hara, Adachi, Ueda, Miyagi, & Enomoto. Risk factors for HPV infection and high-grade cervical disease in sexually active Japanese women.

[19] Ozaydin-Yavuz1, O., Bilgili, S.G., Guducuoglu, H., Yavuz1, I.H., Elibuyuk-Aksac, S., Karadag, A.S. Determinants of high-risk human papillomavirus infection in anogenital warts. Adv Dermatol Allergol 2019; XXXVI (1): 76-81. DOI: https://doi.org/10.5114/ada.2019.82915

[20] Moghadam, O. et al. Infectious Agents and Cancer (2020) 15:52 https://doi.org/10.1186/s13027-020-00318-3

[21] Patel PR, Berenson AB. Sources of HPV vaccine hesitancy in parents. Hum Vaccin Immunother. 2013 Dec;9(12):2649-53. doi: 10.4161/hv.26224. Epub 2013 Aug 27. PMID: 23982270; PMCID: PMC4162068.

[22] Domgue J., Chido-Amajuoyi O.G., Yu R.K., Shete S. (2019). Beliefs About HPV Vaccine's Success at Cervical Cancer Prevention Among Adult US Women. JNCI Cancer Spectr. 2019 Aug27;3(4):pkz064. doi: 10.1093/jncics/pkz064. PMID: ; PMCID: PMC690108

[23] Berenson AB, Hirth JM, Kuo YF, Starkey JM, Rupp RE. Use of patient navigators to increase HPV vaccination rates in a pediatric clinical population. Prev Med Rep. 2020 Aug 28;20:101194. doi: 10.1016/j.pmedr.2020.101194. PMID: 32963935; PMCID: PMC7490555.

[24] Amboree TL, Darkoh C. Barriers to Human Papillomavirus Vaccine Uptake Among Racial/Ethnic Minorities: a Systematic Review. J Racial Ethn Health Disparities. 2020 Oct 6:10.1007/s40615-020-00877-6. doi: 10.1007/s40615-020-00877-6. Epub ahead of print. PMID: 33025422; PMCID: PMC8021610.

Chapter 6

Cervical Cancer Prevention and Control

Tariku Laelago Ersado

Abstract

Cervical cancer is caused by HPV (human papilloma virus). It is the second most common cancer in women living low developed countries. The components of cervical cancer prevention and control comprises primary prevention, secondary prevention and tertiary prevention. Primary prevention of cervical cancer encompasses prevention of infection with HPV. Giving HPV vaccine for girls aged 9–14 years before they initiate sexual activity is one of the interventions of primary prevention of cervical cancer. Screening and treatment is needed in secondary prevention of cervical cancer. Screening of cervical cancer encompasses testing a target group (women) who are at risk for a cervical pre-cancer. Tertiary prevention of cervical cancer comprises treatment of cervical cancer and palliative care. The components of tertiary care comprise surgery, radiotherapy, chemotherapy and palliative care. Community mobilization, health education and counseling on cervical cancer prevention and control is vital to make ownership on cervical prevention. Monitoring and evaluation of cervical cancer prevention and control on key program indicators should be done regularly.

Keywords: cervical cancer, primary prevention, secondary prevention, tertiary prevention, control, vaccination

1. Introduction

Cervical cancer is caused by sexually acquired infection with certain types of HPV (human papilloma virus). HPV is a group of viruses that are extremely common worldwide. There are more than 100 types of HPV, of which at least 14 are cancer-causing [1]. Worldwide, cervical cancer is the fourth most frequent cancer in women. There were 570 000 new cases of cervical in 2018. More than 311 000 deaths from cervical cancer occur every year. More than 85% of these deaths occur in low and middle income countries. Seventy-percent of cervical cancers worldwide are caused by only two HPV types (16 and 18) [1, 2].

Abnormal vaginal bleeding is the common symptom of cervical cancer. The bleeding can occur after sexual intercourse. Bleeding after menopause or increased vaginal discharge may also be symptoms [3].

There are numerous risk factors the can cause cervical cancer. Educational status, place of residence, using old sanitary napkins, younger age at marriage, sexual transmitted infections, number of partners and health service utilization are associated with cervical cancer. Bathing daily and during menstruations is found to be preventive factors for cervical cancer [4, 5]. Women who have HIV infection have an increased risk for cervical cancer than women who have no HIV infection [3, 6]. Non access to cervical cancer screening, commence sexual intercourse at early age, cigarette smoking and long term use of oral contraceptives are also related with higher risk of cervical cancer [3, 5]. History of genital warts, immunosuppression, multiparty, diet low in folates, carotene and vitamin C are also included in risk factors of cervical cancer [7].

The component of cervical cancer prevention and control comprise primary, secondary and tertiary prevention. Cervical cancer can often be prevented by having regular screenings with pap tests and HPV tests to find any pre-cancers and treat them. It can also be prevented by receiving the HPV vaccine [8]. World health organization (WHO) recommended vaccine that can protect HPV 16 and 18 and the vaccine is approved for use in many countries [9]. Avoiding exposure to risk factors is additional actions to prevent cervical cancer [8].

WHO put new cervical elimination targets of 90% HPV vaccination coverage, 70% screening coverage, 90% access to treatment for cervical pre-cancer and cancer and access to palliative care by 2030. Attaining these targets can decrease more than 40% of new cervical cancer cases and 5 million associated mortality by 2050. To achieve this targets efforts should be increased [6]. Availing updated evidence based information on cervical cancer prevention and control is important to increase the information coverage and to develop best strategies that focus on cervical cancer prevention and control. The aim of this chapter is providing the best available information on cervical cancer prevention and control. The chapter described three components of cervical cancer prevention, community mobilization, education and counseling on cervical cancer prevention and monitoring and evaluating cervical cancer prevention and control.

2. Prevention and control of cervical cancer

The goal of any comprehensive cervical cancer prevention and control programme is to decrease the burden of cervical cancer. This can be done by reducing HPV infections, detecting and treating cervical, pre-cancer lesions, and providing timely treatment and palliative care for invasive cancer [9].

The key components of comprehensive cervical cancer prevention and control contains three interdependent components: primary, secondary and tertiary prevention (**Figure 1**). In **Figure 1**, programmatic interventions to prevent HPV infections and cervical cancer is also illustrated.

Even though, effective cervical cancer methods such as HPV vaccination, screening and safe sex practice exists, affordability and putting into practice remain challenge for most countries [5].

Unless cervical cancer prevention and control measures are effectively executed, it is estimated that by 2030, nearly 800,000 new cases of cervical cancer will be annually diagnosed. The huge majority of these cases will be in developing countries [10]. To reduce this burden, community mobilization, education and counseling on cervical cancer prevention should be implemented at all levels. Monitoring and evaluation of cervical cancer prevention and control on key program indicators should also be done on a regular basis.

2.1 Primary prevention of cervical cancer

Prevention of HPV infection is included in primary cervical prevention and control. There are different subtypes of HPV that can cause cervical cancer but, the major subtypes are 16 and 18 [9].

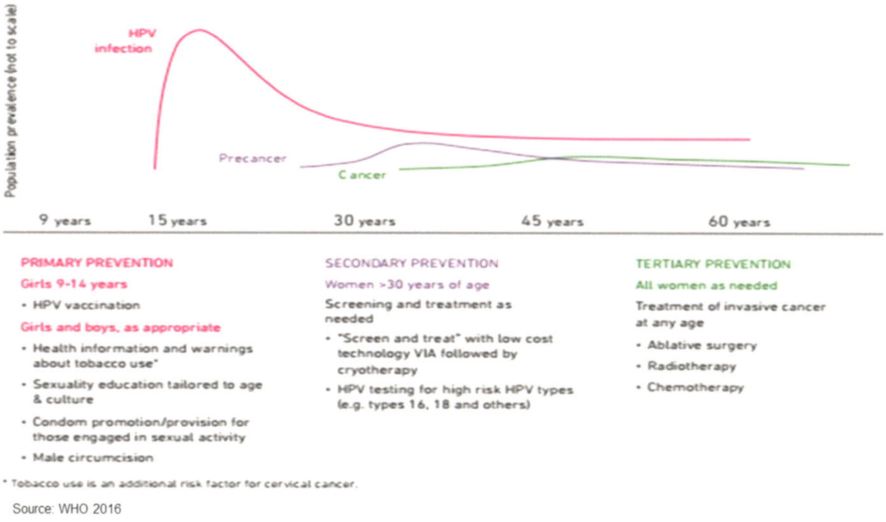

Figure 1.
Programmatic interventions to prevent HPV infections and cervical cancer.

The public health goal of primary prevention of cervical cancer is to reduce HPV infections. Primary prevention can be realized through behavioral change approaches and the use of biological mechanisms, including HPV vaccination. The interventions for primary prevention of cervical cancer include: providing immunization for girls aged 9–14 years before the start sexual intercourse, health education on healthy sexuality for both boys and girls and promotion of condom use. HPV vaccines are not intended to treat women with past or present HPV infection [9, 11].

The target age group for HPV vaccination is 9–14 years earlier to becoming sexual active. Two doses of HPV vaccine with six month interval is required. There is no maximum interval between the two doses. But, the interval of not greater than 12–15 months is suggested to allow girls to complete the schedule on time prior to becoming sexually active. If the interval between doses is shorter than 5 months, then a third dose should be offered at least six months after the first dose. A three dose schedule (at 0, 1–2, and 6 months) is recommended for females 15 years and older and for those known to be immunocompromised and/or HIV-infected [10, 12, 13].

It is not essential to screen for HPV infection or HIV infection prior to HPV immunization. Pre-immunization assessments (e.g., HPV testing of any kind, cervical cancer screening or Pap testing, pregnancy testing, or "virginity testing") are not mandatory [10, 13].

If girls are age ≥ 15 years and received their first dose before age 15 years, they may complete the three doses. If no doses were taken before age 15 years, three doses should be administered. In both scenarios, immunization can be given up to 26 years. If adequate resources remain after immunizing girl's age 9 to 14 years, girls who received one dose may take extra doses between age 15 and 26 years. If there is ≥50% coverage in the priority female target population, sufficient resources and cost effectiveness, boys may be immunized to prevent other non-cervical human papillomavirus related cancers and diseases [12].

The HPV vaccines prevent over 95% of HPV infections caused by HPV types 16 and 18. It may have some cross-protection against other less common HPV types which cause cervical cancer [14]. There are three various vaccines, which vary in the number of HPV types they comprise and target. However, not all are obtainable in everywhere.

- Quadrivalent HPV vaccine (Gardasil®) targets HPV types 6, 11, 16 and 18.
- 9-valent vaccine (Gardasil 9®) targets the same HPV types as the quadrivalent vaccine as well as types 31, 33, 45, 52 and 58.
- Bivalent vaccine (Cervarix ®) targets HPV types 16 and 18 [5].

Cervarix is the best cost effective vaccine with proved efficacy in one dose. The WHO commends two doses for either Gardasil 9 or Cervarix for those up to 15 years of age and three doses for women 15 years or older. The WHO commends are grounded on induced antibody titers at month 7 for Gardasil and Gardasil 9 as there are at present no efficacy data for these vaccines in fewer than three doses. The WHO recommendations for Cervarix are built on efficacy information in addition to immunogenicity information. Three dose efficacy prevents cervical intraepithelial neoplasia (CIN) 2 or worse by any HPV type is around 62% for both Cervarix and Gardsail9. The three dose efficacy prevents CIN 3 or worse by any HPV type is 93% for Cervarix and 43% for Gardasil, with no information for ardasil9 [10, 15] (**Table 1**).

There are numerous HPV vaccination distribution approaches. The followings are commonly used distribution approaches:

- Vaccine distribution at health care facilities
- Vaccine distribution through outreach
- Vaccine distribution through campaigns [9, 10, 16].

Educational interventions announcing the risk of HPV and the benefits of vaccines are important, especially in low and middle income countries [17]. Education and effective communication is vital in attaining successful immunization programme [18].

2.2 Secondary prevention of cervical cancer

In secondary prevention of cervical cancer, screening and treatment as desired is included. Screening comprises testing women who are at risk for a cervical precancer. The aim of screening is to detect and treat those people identified as having early signs of the illness, usually by means of inexpensive, precise, and reliable test that can be practical widely. The other aim of screening is to decrease the death related with cervical cancer through identifying the illness when still at an early treatable stage or through detecting precursor lesions. The systematic removal of CIN lesion during screening also leads to reductions of the incidence of invasive cervical cancers of all stages.

There are numerous cervical cancer screening tests in use or being studied around the world. Cervical cytology has been in use for the past 50 years. Newer screening tests are HPV DNA testing and visual screening tests [19]. Increasing the acceptance of screening has many sigfinaces in preventing cervical cancer through early detection and treatment of pre-cancerous changes before malignancy grows. Approaches of inspiring women to start cervical cancer screening include inviting, reminding, teaching, communication framing, counseling, risk factor identification and financial interventions. Use of invitations and to a lesser degree educational resource are supported by evidence as a good methods of encouraging women to undertaken cervical cancer screening [20].

Attributes	Bivalent(CERVARIX®)	QUADRIVALENT (GARDASIL®/ SILGARD®)	9-VALENT (GARDASIL 9®)
Vaccine	Recombinant L1-capsid virus-like particles (VLP)	Recombinant L1-capsid virus-like particles (VLP)	Recombinant L1-capsid virus-like particles (VLP)
HPV types in vaccine	16,18	6,11,16,18	6,11,16,18 31,33,45,52,58
Disease protection	Cervical cancer (and premalignant genital lesions of cervix, vulva and vagina)	Cervical cancer (and premalignant genital lesions of cervix, vulva and vagina) Genital warts	Cervical cancer (and premalignant genital lesions of cervix, vulva and vagina) Genital warts
Cross-protection against HPV-types	31, 33	31, 45	Not necessary
Number of doses required	2	2	2
Dosing interval (flexibility)	0 and 6 months (No maximum interval but suggested not more than 12–15 months)	0 and 6 months (No maximum interval but suggested not more than 12–15 months)	0 and 6 months (No maximum interval but suggested not more than 12–15 months)
Method of administration	Intramuscular injection	Intramuscular injection	Intramuscular injection
Presentation and Type of Vaccine Vial Monitor (VVM)	1-dose vial; VVM 30 2-dose vial; VVM 30	1-dose vial; VVM 30	1-dose vial; VVM TBD
Shelf-life	48 months at 2–8 °C for 1-dose vial; 36 months at 2–8°C for 2-dose vial; vaccine is freeze sensitive	36 months at 2–8°C, vaccine is freeze sensitive	36 months at 2–8°C, vaccine is freeze sensitive
Contraindications	Severe allergic reaction to any vaccine component after first dose • Severe febrile illness • Known to be pregnant	Severe allergic reaction to any vaccine component after first dose • Severe febrile illness • Known to be pregnant	Severe allergic reaction to any vaccine component after first dose • Severe febrile illness • Known to be pregnant

Source: WHO [10].

Table 1.
Characteristics of HPV vaccines.

Screening of cervical cancer is identifying for pre-cancer. Cervical cancer screening is recommended for woman aged 30 up to 49 years at least one in life time. Early detection and treatment of precancerous lesions can prevent the majority of cervical cancers.

HPV vaccination does not substitute cervical cancer screening. In countries where HPV vaccine is introduced, screening programs may need to be developed or strengthened [21]. Visual inspection of the cervix without magnification was the first technique of screening of the cervix. Nowadays, three types of tests are encouraged:

- Conventional Pap smear (or cytology) and liquid-based cytology
- Visual inspection with Acetic Acid (VIA) or with lugol iodine (VILI)
- HPV testing for high risk HPV types (types 16 and 18).

The randomized trial studies done in different places on cervical cancer screening have shown the efficacy of visual inspection, cytology screening and HPV screening [22–24]. Many studies have acknowledged that in countries where the resources exist to confirm high value and good coverage of the people, cytology screening provides to decreasing the incidence of advanced stage cancers and death related with cervical cancer [25–27].

The treatment methods mostly used are cryotherapy, loop electrosurgical excision procedure or cold-knife conisation [5].

There are two kinds of HPV tests:

- The test that identify if 13 up to 14 HPV subtypes are present or not. But this test cannot help to identify which subtypes are present.
- The tests performed to identify HPV genotyping and identify if HPV 16 or 18 is present or not.

HIV infected women should undergo cervical cancer screening twice in the first year after diagnosis of HIV infection and then annually. For women with two successive normal cytological examinations, the recommendation is that annual follow up includes a detailed visual inspection of the anus, vulva, and vagina, as well as the cervix [5].

Cervical screening based on HPV testing can prevents more invasive cervical cancer and precancerous lesions. It can offers innovative options such as self-collection of specimens to improve screening uptake broadly [28].

2.3 Tertiary prevention of cervical cancer

Tertiary prevention of cervical cancer comprises treatment of cervical cancer and palliative care. Surgical treatment, chemotherapy, radiotherapy and palliative are included in tertiary cervical cancer prevention [16]. The public health goal of tertiary prevention of cervical cancer is to reduce the number of mortality due to cervical cancer.

The interventions for tertiary prevention of cervical cancer comprise:

- A referral mechanism from primary care providers to facilities that offer cancer diagnosis and treatment
- Accurate and timely cancer diagnosis by exploring the extent of invasion
- Treatment, appropriate to each stage based on the diagnosis [9].

2.4 Community mobilization, education and counseling on cervical cancer prevention

Community mobilization is a process of engaging communities and generating support for all those in need of health services, resulting in sustainable community ownership and involvement. Effective communication can increase rates of vaccination and screening and save women's lives. Health care workers and others involved in cervical cancer control at all levels should be trained in basic counseling skills, so that they can communicate effectively with clients. The content of the counseling encounter will vary according to the client's problems or concerns and her individual situations. It can address prevention, screening, follow-up, referral, diagnosis, treatment of precancerous lesions, treatment of invasive cancer and/or palliative care [9].

2.5 Monitoring and evaluating (M & E) cervical cancer prevention and control

Monitoring and assessing the improvement of objectives and targets at country level is crucial. The followings are crucial indicators of cervical cancer preventions and control:

- Immunization coverage by year of age and by dose.
- Screening coverage, screening test positivity rate and treatment rate.
- Proportion of curable cancer patients who get adequate treatment and survival rates.
- Opioid access for women with advanced cervical cancer.

Essential impact indicators of cervical cancer are incidence and death. Establishing cancer register is important to monitor the incidence and death rate of cervical cancer. The register will help to assess long term impacts of cervical cancer screening, treatment and vaccination [21]. The main recording and reporting tools that are used for immunization should be adapted to include HPV vaccine. The recording and reporting tools comprises: immunization register, tally sheet, immunization card, defaulter tracking system, stock record and integrated monthly report [10].

M & E helps the management team to determine the extent to which the program is meeting the stated goals, objectives, targets and make corrections accordingly [16].

An effective program of prevention and control of cervical cancer must address several issues, including the coverage and quality of screening services, availability of diagnosis, treatment and monitoring [29].

Depending on the country setting and resources available, M & E of cervical cancer prevention can be done by using different approaches.

The approaches includes:

- Site visits
- Peer assessment
- Client and community assessment
- Use of new information and communication technology [30].

3. Conclusion

Cervical cancer prevention and control components are primary prevention, secondary prevention and tertiary prevention. Primary prevention comprise HPV vaccination of girls 9–14 years old. Secondary prevention include screening and treatment with low technology VIA followed by cryotherapy. Tertiary prevention of cervical cancer incorporates treatment of invasive cancer and providing palliative care. Mobilizing community, giving health education and counseling is very important in prevention and control of cervical cancer. M & E of cervical cancer prevention and control on key program indicators should also be done regularly.

4. Terminology

Bivalent: a vaccine that works by stimulating an immune response against two different antigens; e.g. Cervarix is a bivalent vaccine that helps protect the body against infection with HPV types 16 and 18.

Chemotherapy: The term that usually describes the use of drugs to treat cancer but which may also describe the use of antibiotics to treat infectious diseases.

Cervical intraepithelial neoplasia (CIN): abnormalities in the cells of the cervix which may become cancerous.

Cryotherapy: the use of cold or freezing in treatment.

Cytology: the study of individual cells. Cytology's main use in medicine is to detect abnormal cells. It is widely used to screen for cancer (as in the cervical smear test) or to confirm a diagnosis of cancer.

DNA (deoxyribonucleic acid): the principal molecule carrying genetic information in almost all organisms.

Immunogenicity: the property of eliciting an immune response.

Neoplasia: the pathological process that results in the formation and growth of a tumor.

Palliative treatment: treatment that relieves the symptoms of a disorder but does not cure it.

Opioid: a type of drug used to relieve strong pain, e.g. morphine.

Quadrivalent: a vaccine that works by stimulating an immune response against four different antigens; e.g. Gardasil is a quadrivalent vaccine that helps protect the body against infection with HPV types 6, 11, 16 and 18.

Screening: The application of a test to people who are as yet asymptomatic for the purpose of classifying them with respect to their likelihood of having a particular disease. It is not undertaken to diagnose a disease, but to identify individuals with increased probability of having either the disease itself or a precursor of the disease.

Prognosis: An assessment of the probable course and outcome of a disease.

DOI: http://dx.doi.org/10.5772/intechopen.99620

Author details

Tariku Laelago Ersado
Department of Nursing, Wachemo University Durame Campus, Durame, Ethiopia

*Address all correspondence to: tarikulalago@gmail.com

References

[1] WHO. Human papillomavirus (HPV) and cervical cancer. 2020.

[2] WHO. human papillomavirus and cervical cance. Available from: https://www.who.int/news-rooms/fact-sheets/detail/human-papillomavirus-(hpv)-and-cervical-cancer WHO; 2019.

[3] American cancer society. Cancer Facts & Figures. American cancer society; 2015.

[4] Kashyap N, Krishnan N, Kaur S, Ghai S. Risk factors of cervical cancer: a case control study. Asia-Pacifc Journal of Oncology Nursing. 2019;6(3):7.

[5] Ngoma M, Autier P. Cancer prevention: cervical cancer. ecancer. 2019;13(952):6.

[6] WHO. WHO releases new estimates of the global burden of cervical cancer associated with HIV. 2020.

[7] Aggarwal P. Cervical cancer: Can it be prevented? World Journal of Clinical Oncology. 2014;5(4):7.

[8] cervical cancer: screening and prevention. http://www.cancer.net. types/cervical-cancer/screening-and-prevention: Cancer. Net; 2020.

[9] WHO. Comprehensive Cervical Cancer Control: A guide to essential practice. Geneva, Switzerland: WHO; 2014.

[10] WHO. Guide to INTRODUCING HPV VACCINE INTO NATIONAL IMMUNIZATION PROGRAMMES. In: Immunization VaB, editor. Geneva: Expanded Programme on Immunization (EPI) 2016. p. 104.

[11] P.Reddi Rani, Reddy KS. Primary Prevention of cerivcal Cancer JPOG MAR/APR. 2016:6.

[12] Silvina Arrossi, Temin S, Garland S, Eckert LON, Bhatla N, † XC, et al. Primary Prevention of Cervical Cancer: American Society of Clinical Oncology Resource-Stratified Guideline. JGO – Journal of Global Oncology. 2017;3(5):24.

[13] Meites E, Gee J, Unger E, Markowitz L. Human Papillomaviruses.

[14] Arbyn M, Xu L, Simoens C, PPL M-H. Prophylactic vaccination against human papillomaviruses to prevent cervical cancer and its precursors Cochrane Database Syst Rev 2018.

[15] Habadi MI, Aljohani HHN, Altayeb MA, Alwosibai HA, Allehyani MAS, Almozain MAM, et al. HUMAN PAPILLOMA VACCINE OVERVIEW. INDO AMERICAN JOURNAL OF PHARMACEUTICAL SCIENCES. 2019;6(2):7.

[16] FMOH. Guideline for Cervical Cancer Prevention and Control in Ethiopia. Adis Ababa: FMOH; 2015. p. 62.

[17] Cheng L, YanWang, Du J. Human Papillomavirus Vaccines: An Updated Review. vaccines. 2020;8(391):15.

[18] Bello F, Enabor O, Adewole I. Human Papilloma Virus Vaccination for Control of Cervical Cancer: A Challenge for Developing Countries. African Journal of Reproductive Health. 2011;15(1):6.

[19] Alliance for Cervical Cancer Prevention. Planning and Implementing Cervical Cancer Prevention and Control Programs: A MANUAL FOR MANAGERS. Alliance for Cervical Cancer Prevention; 2004.

[20] Everett T, Bryant A, Griffin MF, Martin-Hirsch PPL, Forbes CA, RG J. Interventions targeted at women to

encourage the uptake of cervical screening (Review). The Cochrane Collaboration. 2011(5):98.

[21] WHO. WHO GUIDANCE NOTE: Comprehensive cervical cancer prevention and control: a healthier future for girls and women. Switzerland: WHO; 2013.

[22] Van der Aa MA, Pukkala E, Coebergh JW, Anttila A, S S. Mass screening programmes and trends in cervical cancer in Finland and the Netherlands Int J Cancer. 2008;122(8):5.

[23] Sigurdsson K, Sigvaldason H. Longitudinal trends in cervical histological lesions (CIN 2-3+): a 25-year overview Acta Obstet Gynecol Scand. 2006;85(3):6.

[24] Tan N, Sharma M, Winer R, Galloway D, Rees H, RV B. Model-estimated effectiveness of single dose 9-valent HPV vaccination for HIVpositive and HIV-negative females in South Africa. Vaccines. 2018;36:7.

[25] Li X, Stander MP, Van Kriekinge G, N D. Cost-effectiveness analysis of human papillomavirus vaccination in South Africa accounting for human immunodeficiency virus prevalence BMC Infect Dis. 2015;15(566).

[26] Sinanovic E, Moodley J, Barone MA, Mall S, Cleary S, J H. The potential cost-effectiveness of adding a human papillomavirus vaccine to the cervical cancer screening programme in South Africa Vaccine. vaccines. 2009;27(44):7.

[27] Tracy JK, Schluterman NH, Greene C, Sow SO, Gaff HD. Planning for human papillomavirus (HPV) vaccination in sub-Saharan Africa: a modeling-based approach vaccines. 2014;32(26):7.

[28] Ogilvie G, Nakisige C, Huh WK, Mehrotra R, Jeronimo ELF. Optimizing secondary prevention of cervical cancer: Recent advances and future challenges. Int J Gynecol Obstet. 2017;138(1):5.

[29] Manuel V-HV. Screening and Prevention of Cervical Cancer in the World. J Gynecol Res Obstet. 2017; 3(3):7.

[30] WHO, Pan African Health Organization. Monitoring national cervical cancer prevention and control programmes: quality control and quality assurance for visual inspection with acetic acid (VIA)-based programmes. Swizerland WHO, Pan African Health Organization; 2013. p. 41.

Section 4

Treatment and Prognosis

Chapter 7

Insights of Cisplatin Resistance in Cervical Cancer: A Decision Making for Cellular Survival

Elizabeth Mahapatra, Salini Das, Souvick Biswas, Archismaan Ghosh, Debomita Sengupta, Madhumita Roy and Sutapa Mukherjee

Abstract

The clinical scenario of acquired cisplatin resistance is considered as a major impediment in cervical cancer treatment. Bulky drug-DNA adducts formed by cisplatin elicits *DNA damage response (DDR)* which either subsequently induces apoptosis in the cervical cancer cells or enables them to adapt with drug assault by invigorating pro-survival molecular cascades. When HPV infected cervical cancer cells encounter cisplatin, a complex molecular interaction between *deregulated tumor suppressors*, *DNA damage-repair enzymes*, and *prosurvival molecules* get initiated. Ambiguous molecular triggers allow cancer cells to cull apoptosis by opting for a survival fate. Overriding of the apoptotic cues by the pro-survival cues renders a *cisplatin resistant phenotype* in the tumor microenvironment. The present review undrapes the impact of deregulated signaling nexus formed due to crosstalk of the key molecules related to cell survival and apoptosis in orchestrating platinum resistance in cervical cancer.

Keywords: HPV, Cervical cancer, Cisplatin resistance, tumor suppressors, DNA-damage repair, prosurvival signaling

1. Introduction

Cervical cancer, one of the widespread gynecological cancers, accounts for the maximum deaths amongst women across the globe. As per GLOBOCAN 2018, cervical cancer is helmed as the fourth leading cause of mortality and morbidity in women after breast and ovarian cancers [1]. As revealed from the data collated by World Health Organization (WHO) in 2013, over 85% of the cervical cancer cases had surfaced mostly from developing countries with a poor socio-economic backdrop [2]. Women, owing to lack of awareness, often arrive for seeking medical help when the malignant growth of cervix has attained advancement [3].

Infections with a special class of oncogenic DNA viruses called *Human Papilloma Viruses (HPVs)*, hailing from the viral family *Papillomaviridae,* are highly accredited for the malignant transformation of cervix. Principally, HPVs are sexually transmitted [4]. On the basis of its carcinogenic potentials, HPVs can be categorized as –*(i) low-risk HPVs(lr-HPVs)* like *HPV 6, 11, 42, 43* and *44*, and *(ii) high-risk*

IntechOpen

*HPVs(hr-HPVs)*like *HPV 16, 18, 31, 33, 34, 35, 39, 45, 51, 52, 56, 58, 59, 66, 68* and *70* [4, 5]. Persistent and prevalent infections with hr-HPVs contribute in development of cervical cancer alongside other cancers such as the cancer of vagina, vulva, penis, anus, head and neck. HPV infections may also give rise to anogenital warts and recurrent respiratory papillomatosis [5, 6]. Besides HPVs, several other risk factors have been implicated in the etiology of cervical cancer. These mainly include long term use of oral contraceptive [7], smoking [8] and infections with *Chlamydia trachomatis* [9].

Cervical cancer progresses through stages of *mild dysplasia*, *moderate dysplasia* and *severe dysplasia* to finally aggravate into *carcinoma in situ* and *invasive cancer* **stages** [10]. The International Federation of Gynecology and Obstetrics (FIGO) classify these developmental grades of *cervical intraepithelial neoplasia (CIN)* into various stages [11, 12]. Rise in the global disease burden is majorly due to *treatment failure* and *disease recurrence* [13]. The advent of vaccination has allowed for pre-infection protection [14]. However, lack of cost-effectiveness has limited its use to only a certain section of the society, particularly in low income countries like India. The therapeutic modality therefore, is skewed to *chemotherapy* and *radiotherapy*. Stage specific treatment regime is followed for treating cervical cancer [15]. As per FIGO conventions, *Stage IIB-IVA* denotes invasive stages where treatment is ensued in forms of conventional modes of chemotherapy and radiotherapy [11]. Traditionally, chemotherapy involves use of *platinum ligated drugs* like *cisplatin (cis-diamminedichloroplatinum; CDDP)* [16, 17]. Cisplatin in combination with other chemotherapeutics is often employed for treating invasive stages [16]. Patients are often subjected to treatment with cisplatin as a '*radiosensitizer*' prior to radiotherapeutic intervention in the *Concurrent Chemoradiotherapy (CCRT)* regime [16]. Accordingly, cisplatin is the '*drug of choice*' to oncologists for treating cervical cancer irrespective of its different stages.

In the process of HPV mediated cervical carcinogenesis several molecular changes are incited which remodels the metabolic profiles of the cervix [18]. HPV induced metabolic paradigm shift bestows the cells with therapy evasive properties. Consequentially, neoplastic cells emerge as highly dynamic and evolving entities [19]. On encountering drugs, the rewired signaling cascades of the tumor cells residing in the cervix get triggered. These eventuate in increased metabolism of chemotherapeutics like cisplatin, finally catering in reduced intracellular drug accumulation [20], paving a way for acquired cisplatin resistance. This chapter majorly discusses the mechanisms underlying the acquirement of resistance towards cisplatin as a result of deregulated activities of tumor suppressors, DNA damage repair enzymes and prosurvival molecules, mediated due to HPV infections.

2. HPVs: Integral to etiology of cervical cancer

HPVs are relatively small non-enveloped viruses with a diameter of 55 nm. It has a double stranded circular DNA genome which is 8 kb long and is enclosed within an *icosahedral capsid* composed of *72 capsomers* [21, 22]. Functionally, the HPV genome is regionalized into-i) a non-coding regulatory region called the *long control region (LCR)* or the *upper regulatory region (URR)*, ii) an early region which houses *E1, E2, E4, E5, E6* and *E7 genes*, and (iii) a late region which is made up of late expressing genes such as *L1* and *L2* [23]. LCR regulates the process of viral DNA replication via controlling the transcription of Open Reading Frames (ORFs). The lately transcribed proteins L1 and L2 are the structural proteins of the viral capsid. The early genes are dictators of viral replication, transcription, assembly and oncogenesis. Particularly, E6 and E7 are oncogenic and they degrade the cell cycle regulators like p53 and pRb to eventuate in cervical carcinoma [23].

These miniscule infectious agents access the cervical epithelial layer through crevices or microabrasions that generally forms due to mechanical shock or injury. Following entry, HPVs integrate their genome with that of the host to initiate the process of malignant transformation of the cervix (**Figure 1**). The carcinogenesis of cervical epithelium begins with the onset of viral lifecycle which initiates with viral entry into basal cell layer of the epithelium [24]. The basal cell layer of the cervical epidermis enables multiplication and replication of the virus by providing them with a suitable microenvironment. Molecules expressed by the basal cells such as *integrins (α6β1, α6β4), heparan sulphate,* and *proteoglycans* are chemoattractants for HPVs [25, 26]. No sooner does the virus enter the basal cells the viral replication starts but owing to poor copy number the duplication of viral DNA becomes non-reproductive. However, as the infection load spreads into the parabasal and intermediate layers, which are majorly comprised of semi-differentiated cells or terminally differentiated keratinocytes, DNA copy number increases and productive viral replication commences [27]. Meanwhile, the process of cervical carcinogenesis gets driven as the virus multiplies and sustains itself in the host system.

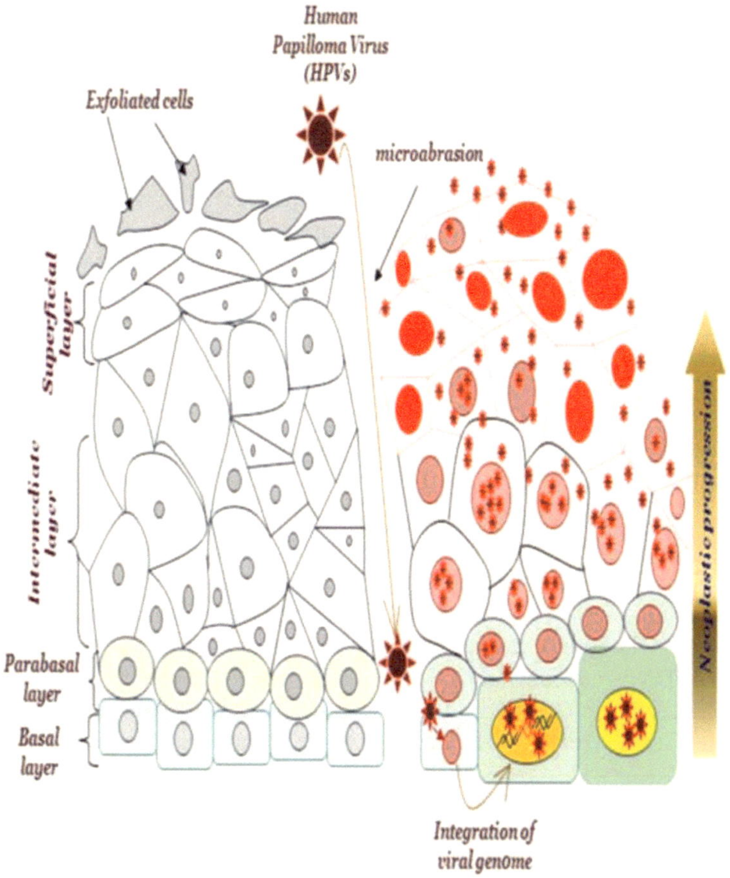

Figure 1.
Host cell hijacking by HPVs. HPVs enter the cervical epithelium through micro abrasions to finally integrate its genome into the DNA of the basal cells to promote loss of genomic integrity. Carcinogenesis is accompanied by viral multiplication in the cervical epithelium.

3. Concomitant molecular changes during cervical carcinogenesis upon HPV infection: an escape route to cisplatin therapy

3.1 Onslaught of HPVs deregulates tumor suppressors

HPV mediated neoplastic transformation of cervix kick starts with the abridgement of tumor suppressor functions. An array of experimentations conducted in *in vitro* and *in vivo* models have successfully established the immortalizing capacities of E6 and E7 viral gene products; ensued via degradation of cell cycle controllers like p53 and pRb [28, 29]. E6 promotes ubiquitin mediated degradation of p53 in assistance with *E6-associated protein (E6AP),* a homolog for *MDM-2* expressed in cells infected with hr-HPVs [30, 31]. As per reports, E6AP very efficaciously reduces the half-life of p53 in HPV infected cervical carcinoma cells, precisely as *MDM-2,* the conventional p53 inhibitor [32]. The guardian of the genome, p53, controls and coordinates the major genetic players involved in *cell cycle arrest* [33]. On top of this, p53 choreographs *DNA damage repair*, and *apoptotic events* [34]. As the episome formation is successfully accomplished by the virus, *DNA damage response (DDR)* is triggered. Absence of functional p53 allows the cervical cells to skip *G1-arrest* [35]. These functions which are central to cell survival and death get violated in the HPV immortalized cervical cells owing to reduced p53 levels. A higher E6 level is inversely proportional to cellular p53 levels [36]. Contrarily, the oncoprotein E7 binds with hypophosphorylated retinoblastoma protein (pRb); releasing the growth promoter E2F from the Rb-E2F complex. E2F translocate to the nucleus to enable expression of genes that drive the infected cells through S-phase of the cell cycle [37]. Cumulative loss of function of both of these tumor suppressors enables the infected cells to progress through G1 and S phases even with genetic errors. Shortfall of repair processes ultimately paves a way for genomic disintegrity to prevail; mediating neoplastic growth. Recent reports suggest that E6 and E7 intervene into the tumor suppressor activity by recruiting methyl groups on their promoter region [38, 39]. These oncogenic viral proteins also methylate *cyclinA1* promoter and deregulate cell cycle progression to mediate tumorigenesis [40].

3.2 Cisplatin insensitivity: a consequence of HPV driven deregulation of tumor suppressors

HPV immortalized cervical cancer cells, especially those at the invasive stages, are subjected to treatment with platinum-ligated drugs like cisplatin. Following its cellular entry, cisplatin transforms into a very strong electrophilic species by hydrolytic activation. Such an activated drug generates an electrophilic attack on cellular nucleophiles like DNA and results in formation of bulky drug-DNA adducts which are beyond repair [41]. Inevitably, cancer cells harboring complex cisplatin modified DNA will be arrested in the G1 phase of the cell cycle particularly; due to generation of DDR response and subsequent activation of p53. Generation of cisplatin-DNA adducts activates *Ataxia Telangiectasia Mutated (ATM) vis a vis ATM- and Rad3-related (ATR)* proteins; culminating into phosphorylation at serine 15 residue and stabilization of p53 [42]. ATR along with various other proteins form an axis of ATR/CHK2/p53/p21; which ultimately mediates apoptosis [43–46]. Therefore, p53 functional status is central to mediation of cisplatin cytotoxicity. This was first demonstrated in a study conducted with small-cell lung cancer cells where adenoviral delivery of p53 sensitized them to cisplatin and resulted in apoptosis [47]. A similar study carried out with ovarian cancer cells, reflected cisplatin induced apoptotic death upon adenovirus mediated delivery of p53 [48]. This tumor suppressor takes up multi-modal routes to facilitate cisplatin-induced cell death. Specifically, p53 increases the susceptibility of cancer cells towards cisplatin by degrading *FLIP*

(FLICE-like inhibitory protein) and by binding with the anti-apoptotic mediator *Bcl-xl* to inactivate its function [49, 50]. It further activates other tumor suppressors like *phosphatase and tensin homolog (PTEN)* to shut down PI3K/Akt pathway [51]. Sometimes, hyperinduction of p53 can disable *AMP-kinase (AMPK)* [52]; thereby forcing the cancer cells to succumb to cisplatin cytotoxicity.

In HPV infected cells, this entire p53 dictated cell-death inducing pathway is compromised owing to functional absence of the tumor suppressors. E6 mediated prior degradation of p53 in cervical cancer cells, unprecedentedly makes them tolerant to the drug. It has been experimentally demonstrated that p53-Bax signaling axis elicited cisplatin induced apoptosis in cervical cancer cells [53]. Even in multiple clinical studies, patients retaining wild-type p53 have been found to respond better to platinum based chemotherapy [54]. Expression patterns of p53 are predictive of success rate of cisplatin treatment in adeno-carcinoma of the uterine cervix [55]. A very recent report has envisaged the contribution of p53 in restoring cisplatin sensitivity in CDDP resistant cervical cancer cells, particularly during combination treatment with doxorubicin [56].

3.3 HPV mediated impairment of DNA repair machinery: an auto-corrector of cisplatin-DNA adducts in cervical cancer

Early genes E1 and E2 drive the process of viral replication in the host by acting as an *origin recognition factor (ORF)* and by imparting helicase [57]. Mostly, the viral replication is dependent upon host cell factors, especially those which are involved in DNA damage repair pathways [58]. Not only HPVs, but other viruses like hepatitis C virus (HCV), Epstein–Barr virus (EBV) and human cytomegalovirus (HCMV) concocts the components of DNA damage repair pathway to survive in the host cells [59, 60]. HPV, while attempting to integrate its genome into the host cell's DNA, incurs DNA damage that eventually evokes DDR.

The host cell has various repair pathways working in a well-knitted fashion to clear off irrelevant mistakes that may arise during the process of DNA replication. Some of these include- *base excision repair (BER), nucleotide excision repair (NER), mismatch repair (MMR)*, *homologous recombination (HR)* and *non-homologous end joining (NHEJ)*. This machinery actively functions to correct errors incorporated in DNA during replication while the cell is gradually traversing through different stages of the cell cycle. In instances of assault to DNA architecture hurled as single strands or double strand breaks, recruitment of ATM or ATR proteins occur at the site of damage. Protein complex comprised of *MRN (MRE11-RAD50-NBS1)* and *Tip60* recognizes and recruits these proteins to the site of damage. ATM phosphorylates a series of downstream effectors which includes *CHK2* and the *histone H2A (H2AX)* to begin with the repair process. For correcting double strand breaks, ATM switches over to HR pathway wherein the process of repair is executed by *breast cancer 1/2 (BRCA1, BRCA2), RAD51* and *Partner and Localizer of BRCA2 (PALB2)* molecules [61–63]. In all cases, p53 is found to be the sole dictator of the process as it allows repair to occur by arresting cells with erroneous DNA.

Cervical cancer cells infected with hr-HPVs exhibit an upregulation of *ATM pathway*. Throughout the viral lifecycle, ATM response is constitutively kept activated owing to phosphorylation of its downstream effectors namely CHK2, NBS1 and BRCA1 [62, 63]. Oncogenic early protein E7 along with higher levels of E1 keeps ATM activity always at a hike. E1, the ORF while imparting helicase action, forms pseudo-viral replication origins which initiate the process of DDR by stalling replication forks [64, 65]. In high-risk HPV infected cervical cells, the candidates of ATM pathway accumulates in the nucleus [66]. The differentiated and undifferentiated cells of the cervical epithelium packed with viral genomes also exhibit an upregulation of homologous recombination factors [67, 68]. Studies with pharmacological inhibitors have further delineated that ATM remains activated all throughout the viral life-cycle. It aids in amplification of viral genome within the differentiated squamous cells [69].

In addition to ATM, HPVs also activate ATR pathway. In HPV infected cells considerably higher levels of *ATR-interacting protein* or *ATRIP* and *DNA topoisomerase 2-binding protein 1* or *TopBP1* were noted [70]. Multiple studies have shown that in cells infected with HPVs has remarkably higher levels of total and phosphorylated forms of ATR as well as its downstream effectors, CHK1 [70]. ATM and ATR pathways provide the virus with an access to the host replicative machinery. E7 destroys Rb along with other related tumor suppressors such as p107 and p130, comprising the family of pocket proteins to control the transit of the cells from G1 phase to S-phase. Moreover, the released E2F translocates to the nucleus and lead to translational activation of the responsive gene, some of which are candidates of DNA damage repair pathways [70].

3.4 HPV seized DNA repair machineries of cervical cancer cells encourages acquired Cisplatin resistance

Upregulated activities of DNA damage repair enzymes empower cervical cancer cells to quickly repair the cisplatin-DNA adducts. Cisplatin generates intrastrand cross-links in the DNA to primarily activate *nucleotide excision repair (NER) system* [71]. It has been proposed that NER prevents apoptosis in cisplatin treated cells via activation of the members of the ATM pathway followed by its recruitment to the site of damage in the DNA. In cervical cancer cells, already activated ATM, immediately starts chewing away drug-DNA adducts; leading to resistance. Over 20 proteins hailing from the *excision repair cross-complementation group 1 (ERCC1)* partake in this process of clearing away the cisplatin-DNA conjugates [72]. At the 5′ site of the bulky cisplatin-DNA lesions, ERCC1 gets co-recruited with ERCC4 for excising away DNA-adducts [73]. In HCA-1R, a cisplatin resistant cervical cancer cell line, an upregulation of ERCC1 expression is recognized. Poor cisplatin responders with locally advanced cervical squamous cell carcinoma exhibit elevated levels of ERCC1 [74]. ERCC1, therefore, is considered as a prognostic biomarker for assessing the survival rate of patients receiving chemotherapy or CCRT [75, 76]. Another evolutionarily conserved DNA repair pathway is *Mismatch Repair (MMR)* pathway which is highly implicated in cisplatin resistance of cervical cancer cells [77]. Amongst the MMR proteins, *MutS homolog 2 (MSH2)* has been identified as a contributor of cisplatin resistance in cervical cancer cells [78]. *Post-meiotic segregation 2 (PMS2),* another key member of the MMR system is found to be negatively correlated with cervical cisplatin resistance [79–82].

3.5 HPV mediated upregulation of prosurvival signaling cascades: Another contributor of cisplatin resistance in cervical cancer

'Abortive infection' often referred to active HPV infection, induces the genesis of both benign and malignant neoplasms of the cervix [83]. The oncogenic viral early gene products initiates cervical carcinogenesis by interacting with the crucial prosurvival signaling cascades of the host cell [84]. Besides abrogating p53 and pRb functions, HPVs opportunistically modulate four important cellular survival pathways by interacting with their upstream effectors such as *growth factor receptor, notch receptor, Ras* along with *phosphatidylinositol 3-kinase subunit C (PI3KCA)* gene which is second messenger activating Akt kinases [85, 86].

3.5.1 Activation of PI3K/Akt signaling

PI3K, particularly was found to be amplified and overtly activated in HPV-induced cervical cancers [87, 88]. The activation of MAPK/ERK in turn alters transcription of multiple genes that are important for regulation of cell-cycle progression and cell proliferation. Thus, activation of PI3K begets in Akt activation via phosphorylation of the protein in most of the HPV infected cancers. HPV16 E6 activates receptor protein tyrosine kinases (RTKs) viz. epidermal growth factor receptor (EGFR), insulin receptor beta and insulin-like growth factor receptor beta; lying upstream of the PI3K/Akt pathway [89]. Activation of Akt results into a series of changes in downstream targets. Akt, furthermore can phosphorylate E6 to promote its ability to interact with 14–3-3σ, an important protein required for carcinogenic progression [90]. A strong association between HPV and surged c-myc expression has been evidenced [91–93]. Reportedly, interaction between E6 and c-myc activates the enzymatic function of *telomerase* [94, 95]. In a clinical study, thirty nine out of 46 cervical cancer specimens evinced phosphorylation of Akt at serine 473 [96]. Akt activation was obtained in about, forty-eight percent of stage Ib2-IIb cervical cancer patients. HPV infection destabilizes the host genome for which mutations may be incurred in PIK3CA gene. Some mutations may be activator mutations accounting in Akt hyperactivation in cervical as well as many other HPV-induced cancers [95]. Oncogenic mutations and translational amplification of PIK3CA gene, switch on PI3K/Akt signaling invigoratingly; driving HPV mediated tumorigenesis.

3.5.2 Activation of mTOR signaling

mTOR kinase functions as a cellular rheostat that amalgamates cellular signaling pathways after sensing growth factor, starvation and energy status. Recently, it has been reported that Akt/mTOR activation occurs immediately after exposure to HPV16 pseudovirions [96]. mTOR activation is frequently observed in cervical squamous cell carcinoma, as well as in most HPV positive head and neck squamous cell carcinomas (HNSCC), and oropharyngeal cancers (OPSCC) [93, 97]. HPV oncoproteins E7 and E6 can chronologically activate AKT through pRb binding and subsequently stimulate mTOR in its complex 1 (mTORC1). These upregulated prosurvival signaling molecules lead to a shift in metabolic paradigm of the cancer cells. When subjected to cisplatin treatment, the HPV infected cervical cancer cells start to metabolize the drug faster than usual. This result in rapid drug efflux and eventually lessens intracellular cisplatin levels to orchestrate cisplatin resistance. Therefore, most cisplatin resistant cervical cancer cells are often characterized by the presence of greater levels of cisplatin efflux pumps [98, 99]. Of late, Li et al. showed in their study that in cisplatin resistant cervical cancer cells with upregulated PI3K/Akt pathway, espouses surged levels of *Lysosome-associated protein transmembrane 4β-35 (LAPTM4B-35)* which is another cisplatin exporter [100, 101].

3.5.3 Activation of the Wnt pathway

Nuclear accumulation of β-catenin due to activation of the canonical Wnt/β-Catenin pathway leads to transcriptional activation of a plethora of proliferative genes. This is highly characteristic to HPV16-positive invasive cancers as well as early dysplastic lesions [102, 103]. This phenomenon of nuclear accumulation of β-catenin positively correlates with progression of cervical cancer [104]. Accordingly, β-catenin was found in higher frequencies within the nucleus of cervical cancer cell line SiHa (bearing integrated HPV16) and HeLa (bearing integrated HPV18) [105]. Lichtig et al. proposed that HPV16 E6 could mechanistically activate Wnt/β-catenin pathway in a p53 independent fashion [106]. β-catenin signaling pathway exhibited a regulatory activity over acquired resistance to cisplatin via upregulation of Bcl-xl [107]. Cisplatin resistance got promoted in neoplasia due to shut down of GSK-3β owing to activation of Wnt/β-catenin signaling [108].

3.5.4 Activation of the Notch pathway

Cellular prosurvival juxtracrine signaling axis involving TGFβ/Notch1 is found to be exhilarated in invasive cervical cancer [109]. As the cervical lesions progressed from intraepithelial lesions III to microinvasive carcinoma, Notch1 translocated from the cytoplasm to the nucleus for ease of function [110]. HPV E6 has been identified as an activator of Notch protein in multiple cervical cancer cell lines [111]. Upregulated activities of notch protein induce stemness in cervical cancer cells, thereby enabling them to evade cisplatin driven cytotoxicity. Inhibition of Notch1was found to revert epithelial to mesenchymal transition (EMT); restoring cisplatin sensitivity [112].

3.5.5 Telomerase activation

Viral oncoprotein E6 escalates human telomerase activity by upregulating its catalytic subunit hTERT or telomerase reverse transcriptase [113, 114]. E6 on being

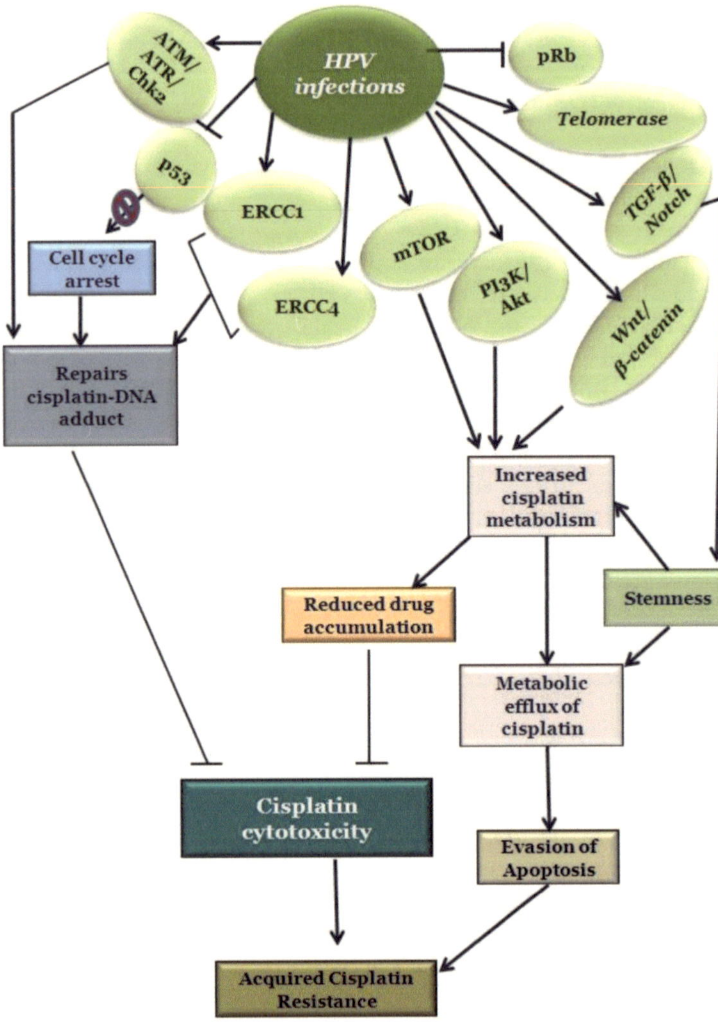

Figure 2.
Concomitant molecular changes induced by HPV contribute in cisplatin resistance in cervical cancer. The viral oncoproteins, particularly E6 and E7 deregulate the crucial molecules involved in cellular metabolism, cell cycle progression, DNA damage repair differentiation, survival, and apoptotic death. These changes provide the cervical cancer cells to evade cytotoxic cell death upon treatment with cisplatin; leading to acquirement of resistance.

aided by E6AP binds to the hTERT promoter region to increase its transcriptional activity [112]. NFX1–123, an mRNA interacting protein gets positively regulated by E6, to maintain higher telomerase expression [115]. E6 upon binding to hTERT protein increases telomerase activity via posttranscriptional modifications [116]. Telomerase reverse transcriptase was reported to promote cisplatin resistance by suppressing apoptosis.

Orchestration of HPV induced signaling nexus in promoting cisplatin resistance in cervical cancer is well depicted in **Figure 2**.

4. Perspective insights

As the virus hijacks the host system, it flips the molecular dynamics according to its own survival benefit. As discussed in this review, loss of function of tumor suppressors, magnified activities of DNA repair enzymes and constitutional activation prosurvival signaling cascades in the HPV infected cervix, make the situation precarious. The conundrum of drug resistance that arises as a result of these existent changes, stymies therapy. Tracking these prior change can aid in planning conventional therapeutic regimes. Thus, these molecules can act as valuable prognostic biomarker before administration of cisplatin based chemotherapy to cervical cancer patients.

Acknowledgements

The authors are indebted to the Director, Chittaranjan National Cancer Institute, Kolkata for encouraging the idea of the manuscript. The authors are grateful to Ministry of Health & Family Welfare, Govt of India for financial support to undertake the research.

Conflict of interest

Authors declare no conflict of interest.

Author details

Elizabeth Mahapatra, Salini Das, Souvick Biswas, Archismaan Ghosh, Debomita Sengupta, Madhumita Roy and Sutapa Mukherjee*
Department of Environmental Carcinogenesis and Toxicology, Chittaranjan National Cancer Institute, Kolkata, India

*Address all correspondence to: sutapa_c_in@yahoo.com

References

[1] Arbyn M, Weiderpass E, Bruni L, de Sanjosé S, Saraiya M, Ferlay J, Bray F. Estimates of incidence and mortality of cervical cancer in 2018: a worldwide analysis. *Lancet Glob Health*. 2020; 8(2): e191-e203.

[2] Bosch FX, Broker TR, Forman D, Moscicki AB, Gillison ML, Doorbar J, Stern PL, Stanley M, Arbyn M, Poljak M, Cuzick J, Castle PE, Schiller JT, Markowitz LE, Fisher WA, Canfell K, Denny LA, Franco EL, Steben M, Kane MA, Schiffman M, Meijer CJ, Sankaranarayanan R, Castellsagué X, Kim JJ, Brotons M, Alemany L, Albero G, Diaz M, de Sanjosé S. Comprehensive control of human papillomavirus infections and related diseases. *Vaccine*. 2013; 31 (7): H1-31.

[3] India State-Level Disease Burden Initiative Cancer Collaborators. The burden of cancers and their variations across the states of India: the Global Burden of Disease Study 1990-2016. *Lancet Oncol*. 2018; 19(10): 1289-1306.

[4] Day PM, Schelhaas M. Concepts of papillomavirus entry into host cells. *Curr Opin Virol*. 2014; 4: 24-31.

[5] De Brot L, Pellegrini B, Moretti ST, Carraro DM, Soares FA, Rocha RM, Baiocchi G, da Cunha IW, de Andrade VP. Infections with multiple high-risk HPV types are associated with high-grade and persistent low-grade intraepithelial lesions of the cervix. *Cancer Cytopathol*. 2017; 125(2): 138-143.

[6] Fortes HR, von Ranke FM, Escuissato DL, Araujo Neto CA, Zanetti G, Hochhegger B, Souza CA, Marchiori E. Recurrent respiratory papillomatosis: A state-of-the-art review. *Respir Med*. 2017; 126: 116-121.

[7] Gierisch JM, Coeytaux RR, Urrutia RP, Havrilesky LJ, Moorman PG, Lowery WJ, Dinan M, McBroom AJ, Hasselblad V, Sanders GD, Myers ER. Oral contraceptive use and risk of breast, cervical, colorectal, and endometrial cancers: a systematic review. *Cancer Epidemiol Biomarkers Prev*. 2013; 22(11): 1931-43.

[8] Puleo GE, Borger TN, Montgomery D, Rivera Rivera JN, Burris JL. A Qualitative Study of Smoking-Related Causal Attributions and Risk Perceptions in Cervical Cancer Survivors. *Psychooncology*. 2020; 29(3): 500-506.

[9] Zhu H, Shen Z, Luo H, Zhang W, Zhu X. *Chlamydia trachomatis* Infection-Associated Risk of Cervical Cancer: A Meta-Analysis. *Medicine(Baltimore)*. 2016; 95(13):e3077.

[10] Jain MA, Limaiem F. Cervical Intraepithelial Squamous Cell Lesion. *Treasure Island (FL): StatPearls Publishing*; 2021.

[11] Bhatla N, Berek JS, Cuello Fredes M, Denny LA, Grenman S, Karunaratne K, Kehoe ST, Konishi I, Olawaiye AB, Prat J, Sankaranarayanan R, Brierley J, Mutch D, Querleu D, Cibula D, Quinn M, Botha H, Sigurd L, Rice L, Ryu HS, Ngan H, Mäenpää J, Andrijono A, Purwoto G, Maheshwari A, Bafna UD, Plante M, Natarajan J. Revised FIGO staging for carcinoma of the cervix uteri. *Int J Gynaecol Obstet*. 2019; 145(1): 129-135.

[12] Ayhan A, Aslan K, Bulut AN, Akilli H, Öz M, Haberal A, Meydanli MM. Is the revised 2018 FIGO staging system for cervical cancer more prognostic than the 2009 FIGO staging system for women previously staged as IB disease? *Eur J Obstet Gynecol Reprod Biol*. 2019; 240: 209-214.

[13] Zhu H, Luo H, Zhang W, Shen Z, Hu X, Zhu X. Molecular mechanisms of cisplatin resistance in cervical

cancer. *Drug Des Devel Ther.* 2016 ; 10: 1885-95.

[14] Sankaranarayanan R, Basu P, Kaur P, Bhaskar R, Singh GB, Denzongpa P, Grover RK, Sebastian P, Saikia T, Oswal K, Kanodia R, Dsouza A, Mehrotra R, Rath GK, Jaggi V, Kashyap S, Kataria I, Hariprasad R, Sasieni P, Bhatla N, Rajaraman P, Trimble EL, Swaminathan S, Purushotham A. Current status of human papillomavirus vaccination in India's cervical cancer prevention efforts. *Lancet Oncol*. 2019; 20(11): e637-e644.

[15] Tsikouras P, Zervoudis S, Manav B, Tomara E, Iatrakis G, Romanidis C, Bothou A, Galazios G. Cervical cancer: screening, diagnosis and staging. *J BUON*. 2016; 21(2): 320-5.

[16] Rogers L, Siu SS, Luesley D, Bryant A, Dickinson HO. Radiotherapy and chemoradiation after surgery for early cervical cancer. *Cochrane Database Syst Rev.* 2012; 5(5): CD007583.

[17] Xiang M, Kidd EA. Benefit of Cisplatin with Definitive Radiotherapy in Older Women with Cervical Cancer. *J Natl Compr Canc Netw*. 2019; 17(8): 969-975.

[18] Ding Z, Yang X, Chernenko G, Tang SC, Pater A. Human papillomavirus type 16-immortalized endocervical cells selected for resistance to cisplatin are malignantly transformed and have a multidrug resistance phenotype. *Int J Cancer*. 2000; 87(6): 818-23.

[19] Navin N, Kendall J, Troge J, Andrews P, Rodgers L, McIndoo J, Cook K, Stepansky A, Levy D, Esposito D, Muthuswamy L, Krasnitz A, McCombie WR, Hicks J, Wigler M. Tumour evolution inferred by single-cell sequencing. *Nature*. 2011; 472(7341): 90-4.

[20] Martinho O, Pinto F, Granja S, Miranda-Gonçalves V, Moreira MA, Ribeiro LF, di Loreto C, Rosner MR, Longatto-Filho A, Reis RM. RKIP inhibition in cervical cancer is associated with higher tumor aggressive behavior and resistance to cisplatin therapy. *PLoS One*. 2013; 8(3): e59104.

[21] Favre M. Structural polypeptides of rabbit, bovine, and human papillomaviruses. *J Virol*. 1975; 15(5): 1239-1247.

[22] Baker TS, Newcomb WW, Olson NH, et al. Structures of bovine and human papillomaviruses. Analysis by cryoelectron microscopy and three dimensional image reconstruction. *Biophys J.* 1991; 60(6): 1445-1456.

[23] Burd EM. Human papillomavirus and cervical cancer. *Clin Microbiol Rev*. 2003; 16(1): 1-17.

[24] Doorbar J, Egawa N, Griffin H, Kranjec C, Murakami I. Human papillomavirus molecular biology and disease association. *Rev Med Virol*. 2015; 25(1): 2-23.

[25] Evander M, Frazer IH, Payne E, Qiy YM, Hengst K, McMillan NA. Identification of the alpha6 integrin as a candidate receptor for papillomaviruses. *J Virol*. 1997; 71(3): 2449-2456.

[26] Giroglou T, Florin L, Schäfer F, Streeck RE, Sapp M. Human papillomavirus infection requires cell surface heparan sulfate. *J Virol*. 2001; 75(3): 1565-70.

[27] Flores ER, Allen-Hoffmann BL, Lee D, Sattler CA, Lambert PF. Establishment of the human papillomavirus type 16 (HPV-16) life cycle in an immortalized human foreskin keratinocyte cell line. *Virology.* 1999; 262(2): 344-54.

[28] Munger K, Howley PM: Human papillomavirus immortalization and transformation functions. *Virus Res*. 2002; 89:213-228.

[29] Howley PM, Scheffner M, Munger K: Oncoproteins encoded by the cancer-associated papillomavirus target the products of retinoblastoma and p53 tumor suppressor genes. *Quant Biol.* 1991; 56: 159-155.

[30] Henstermann A, Linares LK, Ciechanover A: Complete switch from Mdm2 to human papillomavirus E6-mediated degradation of p53 in cervical cancer cells. *Proc Natl Acad Sci USA*. 2001; 98: 1218-1223.

[31] Mantovani F, Banks L: The human papillomavirus E6 protein and its contribution to malignant progression. *Oncogene*. 2001; 20: 7874-7887.

[32] Werness BA, Levine AJ, Howley PM: Association of human papillomavirus types 16 and 18 E6 proteins with p53. *Science*. 1990; 248: 76-79.

[33] Di Leonardo A, Linke SP, Clarkin K, Wahl GM. DNA damage triggers a prolonged p53-dependent G1 arrest and long-term induction of Cip1 in normal human fibroblasts. *Genes Dev*. 1994; 8: 2540-2551.

[34] Smith ML, Chen IT, Zhan Q, O'Connor PM, Fornace AJ Jr. Involvement of the p53 tumor suppressor in repair of u.v.-type DNA damage. *Oncogene.* 1995; 10: 1053-1059.

[35] Thomas M, Pim D, Banks L. The role of the E6-p53 interaction in the molecular pathogenesis of HPV. *Oncogene.* 1999; 18(53): 7690-7700.

[36] Hwang ES, Riese DJ 2nd, Settleman J, Nilson LA, Honig J, Flynn S, DiMaio D: Inhibition of cervical carcinoma cell line proliferation by the introduction of a bovine papillomavirus regulatory gene. *Virology.* 1993; 67: 3720-3729.

[37] Syrj€anen SM, Syrj€anen KJ. New concepts on the role of human papillomavirus in cell cycle regulation. *Ann Med.* 1999; 31(3): 175-187.

[38] Sen P, Ganguly P, Ganguly N. Modulation of DNA methylation by human papillomavirus E6 and E7 oncoproteins in cervical cancer. *Oncol Lett*. 2018;15: 11-22.

[39] Yin F, Wang N, Wang S, Yu F, Sun X, Yu X, Luo B, Zhao C , Wang Y. HPV16 oncogenes E6 or/and E7 may influence the methylation status of RASSFIA gene promoter region in cervical cancer cell line HT-3. *Oncol Rep*. 2017; 37: 2324-2334.

[40] Yanatatsaneejit P, Mutirangura A, Kitkumthorn N. Human papillomavirus's physical state and cyclin A1 promoter methylation in cervical cancer. *Int J Gyneco.* 2011; 21: 902-906.

[41] Eastman A. The formation, isolation and characterization of DNA adducts produced by anticancer platinum complexes. *Pharmacology and Therapeutics*. 1987; 34 (2): 155-166.

[42] Efeyan A, Serrano M. p53: guardian of the genome and policeman of the oncogenes. *Cell Cycle*. 2007; 6(9): 1006-1010.

[43] Pabla N., Huang S., Mi QS, Daniel R, Dong Z. ATRChk2 signaling in p53 activation and DNA damage response during cisplatin-induced apoptosis. *Journal of Biological Chemistry. 2008,* 283(10): 6572-6583.

[44] Kondo S, Barna BP, Kondo Y, Tanaka Y, Casey G, Liu J, Morimura T, Kaakaji R, Peterson JW, Werbel B, Barnett GH. WAF1/CIP1 increases the susceptibility of p53 non-functional malignant glioma cells to cisplatin-induced apoptosis. *Oncogene*. 1996; 13(6): 1279-85.

[45] Zamble DB, Jacks T, Lippard SJ. p53-Dependent and -independent responses to cisplatin in mouse testicular teratocarcinoma cells. *Proc Natl Acad Sci U S A*. 1998; 95(11): 6163-8.

[46] Yang X, Fraser M, Moll UM, Basak A, Tsang BK. Akt-mediated cisplatin resistance in ovarian cancer: modulation of p53 action on caspase-dependent mitochondrial death pathway. *Cancer Res.* 2006; 66(6): 3126-36.

[47] Fujiwara T, Grimm EA, Mukhopadhyay T, Zhang WW, Owen-Schaub LB, Roth JA. Induction of chemosensitivity in human lung cancer cells in vivo by adenovirus-mediated transfer of the wild-type p53 gene. *Cancer Res*. 1994; 54(9): 2287-91.

[48] Kanamori Y, Kigawa J, Minagawa Y, Irie T, Oishi T, Shimada M, Takahashi M, Nakamura T, Sato K, Terakawa N. A newly developed adenovirus-mediated transfer of a wild-type p53 gene increases sensitivity to cis-diamminedichloroplatinum (II) in p53-deleted ovarian cancer cells. *Eur J Cancer*. 1998; 34(11): 1802-6.

[49] Persons DL, Yazlovitskaya EM, Pelling JC. Effect of extracellular signal-regulated kinase on p53 accumulation in response to cisplatin. *J Biol Chem*. 2000; 275(46): 35778-85.

[50] Abedini MR, Muller EJ, Bergeron R, Gray DA, Tsang BK. Akt promotes chemoresistance in human ovarian cancer cells by modulating cisplatin-induced, p53-dependent ubiquitination of FLICE-like inhibitory protein. *Oncogene*. 2010; 29(1): 11-25.

[51] Kutuk O, Arisan ED, Tezil T, Shoshan MC, Basaga H. Cisplatin overcomes Bcl-2-mediated resistance to apoptosis via preferential engagement of Bak: critical role of Noxa-mediated lipid peroxidation. *Carcinogenesis.* 2009; 30(9): 1517-27.

[52] Yan X, Fraser M, Qiu Q, Tsang BK. Over-expression of PTEN sensitizes human ovarian cancer cells to cisplatin-induced apoptosis in a p53-dependent manner. *Gynecol Oncol*. 2006; 102(2): 348-55.

[53] Sultana H, Kigawa J, Kanamori Y, Itamochi H, Oishi T, Sato S, Kamazawa S, Ohwada M, Suzuki M, Terakawa N. Chemosensitivity and p53-Bax pathway-mediated apoptosis in patients with uterine cervical cancer. *Ann Oncol.* 2003; 14(2): 214-9.

[54] Garzetti GG, Ciavattini A, Provinciali M, Di Stefano G, Lucarini G, Goteri G, Biagini G. Expression of p53 and apoptosis of tumor cells in locally advanced cervical carcinoma after cisplatin based neoadjuvant chemotherapy. *Anticancer Res*. 1996; 16(5B): 3229-34.

[55] Saito T, Takehara M, Tanaka R, Lee R, Horie M, Wataba K, Ito E, Kudo R. Correlation between responsiveness of neoadjuvant chemotherapy and apoptosis-associated proteins for cervical adenocarcinoma. *Gynecol Oncol*. 2004; 92(1): 284-92.

[56] Yi SA, Kim GW, Yoo J, Han JW, Kwon SH. HP1γ Sensitizes Cervical Cancer Cells to Cisplatin through the Suppression of UBE2L3. *Int J Mol Sci.* 2020; 21(17): 5976.

[57] Frattini, MG, Laimins, LA. Binding of the human papillomavirus E1 origin-recognition protein is regulated through complex formation with the E2 enhancer-binding protein. *Proc. Natl Acad. Sci. USA*. 1994; 91: 12398-12402.

[58] Sedman J, Stenlund A. Co-operative interaction between the initiator E1 and the transcriptional activator E2 is required for replicator specific DNA replication of bovine papillomavirus in vivo and in vitro. *EMBO J*. 1995; 14: 6218-6228.

[59] Stracker TH, Carson CT, Weitzman MD, Adenovirus oncoproteins inactivate the Mre11-Rad50-NBS1DNA repair complex. *Nature*. 2002; 418: 348-352.

[60] Machida K, McNamara G, Cheng KT, Huang J, Wang, CH,

Comai L, Ou JH, Lai MM. Hepatitis C virus inhibits DNA damage repair through reactive oxygen and nitrogen species and by interfering with the ATM-NBS1/Mre11/Rad50 DNA repair pathway in monocytes and hepatocytes. *J. Immunol.* 2010; 185: 6985-6998.

[61] Hollingworth R, Grand RJ. Modulation of DNA damage and repair pathways by human tumour viruses. *Viruses*. 2015; 7(5):2542-91.

[62] Sy SM, Huen MS, Chen J. PALB2 is an integral component of the BRCA complex required for homologous recombination repair. *Proc Natl Acad Sci U S A*. 2009; 106 (17):7155-60.

[63] Helena JM, Joubert AM, Grobbelaar S, Nolte EM, Nel M, Pepper MS, Coetzee M, Mercier AE. Deoxyribonucleic Acid Damage and Repair: Capitalizing on Our Understanding of the Mechanisms of Maintaining Genomic Integrity for Therapeutic Purposes. *Int J Mol Sci*. 2018; 19(4):1148.

[64] Moody CA, Laimins LA. Human papillomaviruses activate the ATM DNA damage pathway for viral genome amplification upon differentiation. *PLoS Pathog*. 2009; 5.

[65] Sakakibara N, Mitra R, McBride AA. The papillomavirus E1 helicase activates a cellular DNA damage response in viral replication foci. *J. Virol*. 2011; 85: 8981-8995.

[66] Kadaja, M, Isok-Paas, H, Laos T, Ustav, E, Ustav M. Mechanism of genomic instability in cells infected with the high-risk human papillomaviruses. *PLoS Pathog*. 2009; 5.

[67] Gillespie KA, Mehta KP, Laimins LA, Moody CA. Human papillomaviruses recruit cellular DNA repair and homologous recombination factors to viral replication centers. *J. Virol*. 2012; 86: 9520-9526.

[68] McKinney CC, Hussmann KL, McBride AA. The role of the DNA damage response throughout the papillomavirus life cycle. *Viruses.* 2015; 7: 2450-2469.

[69] Hong S, Dutta A, Laimins LA. The acetyltransferase Tip60 is a critical regulator of the differentiation-dependent amplification of human papillomaviruses. *J Virol*. 2015; 89(8): 4668-75.

[70] Bristol ML, Das D, Morgan IM. Why Human Papillomaviruses Activate the DNA Damage Response (DDR) and How Cellular and Viral Replication Persists in the Presence of DDR Signaling. *Viruses.* 2017; 9(10): 268.

[71] Reinson T.; Toots, M.; Kadaja, M.; Pipitch, R.; Allik, M.; Ustav, E.; Ustav, M. Engagement of the ATR-dependent DNA damage response at the human papillomavirus 18 replication centers during the initial amplification. *J. Virol.* 2013; 87: 951-964.

[72] Hong, S.; Cheng, S.; Iovane, A.; Laimins, L.A. STAT-5 regulates transcription of the topoisomerase II beta-binding protein 1 (TopBP1) gene to activate the ATR pathway and promote human papillomavirus replication. *Am. Soc. Microbiol*. 2015; 6.

[73] Boyer, S.N.; Wazer, D.E.; Band, V. E7 protein of human papilloma virus-16 induces degradation of retinoblastoma protein through the ubiquitin-proteasome pathway. *Cancer Res*. 1996; 56: 4620-4624.

[74] Welsh C, Day R, McGurk C, Masters JRW, Wood RD, K¨oberle B. Reduced levels of XPA, ERCC1 and XPF DNA repair proteins in testis tumor cell lines. *International Journal of Cancer.* 2004; 110(3): 352-361.

[75] Martin LP, Hamilton TC, Schilder RJ. Platinum resistance: the role of DNA repair pathways. *Clin Cancer Res*. 2008; 14(5): 1291-1295.

[76] Galluzzi L, Senovilla L, Vitale I, et al. Molecular mechanisms of cisplatin resistance. Oncogene. 2012;31(15):1869-1883.

[77] Torii Y, Kato R, Minami Y, Hasegawa K, Fujii T, Udagawa Y. ERCC1 expression and chemosensitivity in uterine cervical adenocarcinoma cells. *Anticancer Res.* 2014; 34(1): 107-115.

[78] Park JS, Jeon EK, Chun SH, et al. ERCC1 (excision repair cross-complementation group 1) expression as a predictor for response of neoadjuvant chemotherapy for FIGO stage 2B uterine cervix cancer. *Gynecol Oncol*. 2011; 120(2): 275-279.

[79] Hasegawa K, Kato R, Torii Y, Ichikawa R, Oe S, Udagawa Y. The relationship between ERCC1 expression and clinical outcome in patients with FIGO stage I to stage II uterine cervical adenocarcinoma. *Int J Gynecol Cancer*. 2011; 21(8): 1479-1485.

[80] Guthrie OW, Li-Korotky HS, Durrant JD, Balaban C. Cisplatin induces cytoplasmic to nuclear translocation of nucleotide excision repair factors among spiral ganglion neurons. *Hearing Research*. 2008 ; 239(2): 79-91.

[81] Zhang Y, Shu YM, Wang SF, Da BH, Wang ZH, Li HB. Stabilization of mismatch repair gene PMS2 by glycogen synthase kinase 3beta is implicated in the treatment of cervical carcinoma. *BMC Cancer*. 2010; 10: 58.

[82] Doorbar J. The papillomavirus life cycle. *J Clin Virol*. 2005; 32 (1): S7-15.

[83] Burd EM. Human papillomavirus and cervical cancer. *Clin Microbiol Rev*. 2003; 16(1): 1-17.

[84] Keysar SB, Astling DP, Anderson RT, Vogler BW, Bowles DW, Morton JJ, Paylor JJ, Glogowska MJ, Le PN, Eagles-Soukup JR, Kako SL, Takimoto SM, Sehrt DB, Umpierrez A, Pittman MA, Macfadden SM, Helber RM, Peterson S, Hausman DF, Said S, Leem TH, Goddard JA, Arcaroli JJ, Messersmith WA, Robinson WA, Hirsch FR, Varella-Garcia M, Raben D, Wang XJ, Song JI, Tan AC, Jimeno A. A patient tumor transplant model of squamous cell cancer identifies PI3K inhibitors as candidate therapeutics in defined molecular bins. *Mol Oncol*. 2013; 7(4): 776-90.

[85] Lechner M, Frampton GM, Fenton T, Feber A, Palmer G, Jay A, Pillay N, Forster M, Cronin MT, Lipson D, Miller VA, Brennan TA, Henderson S, Vaz F, O'Flynn P, Kalavrezos N, Yelensky R, Beck S, Stephens PJ, Boshoff C. Targeted next-generation sequencing of head and neck squamous cell carcinoma identifies novel genetic alterations in HPV+ and HPV- tumors. *Genome Med*. 2013; 5(5): 49.

[86] Wu J, Chen J, Zhang L, Masci PP, Zhao KN. Four major factors regulate phosphatidylinositol 3-kinasesignaling pathway in cancers induced by infection of human Papillomaviruses. *Curr Med Chem.* 2014; 21 (26): 3057-69.

[87] Lee CM, Fuhrman CB, Planelles V, Peltier MR, Gaffney DK, Soisson AP, Dodson MK, Tolley HD, Green CL, Zempolich KA. Phosphatidylinositol 3-kinase inhibition by LY294002 radiosensitizes human cervical cancer cell lines. *Clin Cancer Res*. 2006; 12(1): 250-6.

[88] Choi SK, Hong YO, Lee WM, Kim EK, Joo JE, Kim DW, Lee H. Overexpression of PI3K-p110α in the progression of uterine cervical neoplasia and its correlation with pAkt and DJ-1. *Eur J Gynaecol Oncol.* 2015; 36(4):389-93.

[89] Spangle JM, Munger K. The HPV16 E6 oncoprotein causes prolonged

receptor protein tyrosine kinase signaling and enhances internalization of phosphorylated receptor species. *PLoS Pathogens*. 2013; 9: e1003237.

[90] McFarlane M, Graham SV. Human papillomavirus regulation of SR proteins. *Biochem Soc Trans.* 2010; 38(4): 1116-21.

[91] Boon SS, Banks L. High-risk human papillomavirus E6 oncoproteins interact with 14-3-3ζ in a PDZ binding motif dependent manner. *Journal of Virology.* 2013; 87: 1586-1595.

[92] Hurlin P, Foley K, Ayer D, Eisenman R, Hanahan D, Arbeit J. Regulation of Myc and Mad during epidermal differentiation and HPV-associated tumorigenesis. *Oncogene*. 1995; 11: 2487-2501.

[93] Dellas A, Schultheiss E, Leivas M, Moch H, Torhorst J. Association of p27Kip1, cyclin E and c-myc expression with progression and prognosis in HPV-positive cervical neoplasms. *Anticancer Research*. 1997; 18: 3991-3998.

[94] DeFilippis RA, Goodwin EC, Wu L, DiMaio D. Endogenous human papillomavirus E6 and E7 proteins differentially regulate proliferation, senescence, and apoptosis in HeLa cervical carcinoma cells. *Journal of Virology*. 2003; 77: 1551-1563.

[95] Veldman T, Liu X, Yuan H, Schlegel R. Human papillomavirus E6 and Myc proteins associate in vivo and bind to and cooperatively activate the telomerase reverse transcriptase promoter. *Proceedings of the National Academy of Sciences*. 2003; 100: 8211-8216.

[96] Menges CW, Baglia LA, Lapoint R, McCance DJ. Human papillomavirus type 16 E7 up-regulates AKT activity through the retinoblastoma protein. *Cancer Res*. 2006; 66(11):5555-9.

[97] Surviladze Z, Sterk RT, Deharo SA, Ozbun MA. Cellular entry of human papillomavirus type 16 involves activation of the phosphatidylinositol 3-Kinase/Akt/mTOR pathway and inhibition of autophagy. *J Virol*. 2013; 87(5):2508-17.

[98] Sewell A, Brown B, Biktasova A, Mills GB, Lu Y, Tyson DR, et al. Reverse-phase protein array profiling of oropharyngeal cancer and significance of PIK3CA mutations in HPV-associated head and neck cancer. *Clin Cancer Res.* 2014;20(9):2300-11.

[99] Roy M, Mukherjee S. Reversal of resistance towards cisplatin by curcumin in cervical cancer cells. *Asian Pac J Cancer Prev*. 2014;15(3): 1403-1410.

[100] Meng F, Tan S, Liu T, Song H, Lou G. Predictive significance of combined LAPTM4B and VEGF expression in patients with cervical cancer. *Tumour Biol*. 2015.

[101] Li L, Wei XH, Pan YP, et al. LAPTM4B: a novel cancer-associated gene motivates multidrug resistance through efflux and activating PI3K/AKT signaling. *Oncogene*. 2010; 29(43):5785-5795.

[102] Pereira-Suárez AL, Meraz MA, Lizano M, Estrada-Chávez C, Hernández F, Olivera P, Pérez E, Padilla P, Yaniv M, Thierry F, García-Carrancá A. Frequent alterations of the beta-catenin protein in cancer of the uterine cervix. *Tumour Biol.* 2002; 23(1): 45-53.

[103] Fadare O, Reddy H, Wang J, Hileeto D, Schwartz PE, Zheng W. E-cadherin and β-catenin expression in early stage cervical carcinoma: a tissue microarray study of 147 cases. *World Journal of Surgical Oncology.* 2005; 3: 38.

[104] Shinohara A, Yokoyama Y, Wan X, Takahashi Y, Mori Y, Takami T,

Shimokawa K, Tamaya T. Cytoplasmic/nuclear expression without mutation of exon 3 of the beta-catenin gene is frequent in the development of the neoplasm of the uterine cervix. *Gynecol Oncol*. 2001; 82(3): 450-5.

[105] Rampias T, Boutati E, Pectasides E, Sasaki C, Kountourakis P, Weinberger P, Psyrri A. Activation of Wnt signaling pathway by human papillomavirus E6 and E7 oncogenes in HPV16-positive oropharyngeal squamous carcinoma cells. *Mol Cancer Res*. 2010; 8(3): 433-43.

[106] Lichtig H, Gilboa DA, Jackman A, Gonen P, Levav-Cohen Y, Haupt Y, Sherman L. HPV16 E6 augments Wnt signaling in an E6AP-dependent manner. *Virology*. 2010; 396(1): 47-58.

[107] Zhang J, Liu J, Li H, Wang J. β-Catenin signaling pathway regulates cisplatin resistance in lung adenocarcinoma cells by upregulating Bcl-xl. *Mol Med Rep*. 2016; 13(3): 2543-2551.

[108] Zhong Z, Virshup DM. Wnt Signaling and Drug Resistance in Cancer. *Mol Pharmacol*. 2020; 97(2): 72-89.

[109] Zagouras P, Stifani S, Blaumueller CM, Carcangiu ML, Artavanis-Tsakonas S. Alterations in Notch signaling in neoplastic lesions of the human cervix. *Proceedings of the National Academy of Sciences*. 1995; 92: 6414-6418

[110] Daniel B, Rangarajan A, Mukherjee G, Vallikad E, Krishna S. The link between integration and expression of human papillomavirus type 16 genomes and cellular changes in the evolution of cervical intraepithelial neoplastic lesions. *Journal of General Virology*. 1997; 78: 1095-1101.

[111] Zhang Y, Koneva LA, Virani S, Arthur AE, Virani A, Hall PB, Warden CD, Carey TE, Chepeha DB, Prince ME, McHugh JB, Wolf GT, Rozek LS, Sartor MA. Subtypes of HPV-Positive Head and Neck Cancers Are Associated with HPV Characteristics, Copy Number Alterations, PIK3CA Mutation, and Pathway Signatures. *Clin Cancer Res*. 2016; 22(18): 4735-45.

[112] Zeng D, Liang YK, Xiao YS, Wei XL, Lin HY, Wu Y, Bai JW, Chen M, Zhang GJ. Inhibition of Notch1 reverses EMT and chemoresistance to cisplatin via direct downregulation of MCAM in triple-negative breast cancer cells. *Int J Cancer*. 2020; 147(2): 490-504.

[113] Klingelhutz AJ, Foster SA, McDougall JK. Telomerase activation by the E6 gene product of human papillomavirus type 16. *Nature*. 1996; 380(6569): 79-82.

[114] Veldman T, Horikawa I, Barrett JC, Schlegel R. Transcriptional activation of the telomerase hTERT gene by human papillomavirus type 16 E6 oncoprotein. *Journal of Virology*. 2001; 75: 4467-4472.

[115] Vliet-Gregg PA, Hamilton JR, Katzenellenbogen RA. NFX1-123 and human papillomavirus 16E6 increase notch expression in keratinocytes. *Journal of Virology*. 2013; 87: 13741-13750.

[116] Liu X, Dakic A, Zhang Y, Dai Y, Chen R, Schlegel R. HPV E6 protein interacts physically and functionally with the cellular telomerase complex. *Proc Natl Acad Sci U S A*. 2009; 106(44): 18780-5.

Section 5

HPV and Carcinogenesis

Chapter 8

Human Papillomavirus and Cervical Cancer

Saliha Sağnıç

Abstract

Cervical cancer is one of the leading female cancers especially in developing countries and a common cause of death among middle-aged women. The main role of Human Papillomavirus (HPV) in both cervical cancer and pre-invasive lesions of the cervix has been proven in studies. Reducing the incidence of the disease can be achieved by the regular cervical screening of women and vaccination of appropriate age groups. The disease can be better controlled by better elucidating the details of HPV carcinogenesis, the interaction between the host and the virus, and determinants of the systemic and cellular immune response to the viral infection. HPV causes oropharyngeal and anogenital diseases in both men and women and is usually sexually transmitted. Most infections are transient and could be cleared spontaneously by the host immune system. After the first encounter with HPV infection, it takes years to progress to cervical cancer, which gives clinicians a long period to follow these patients in terms of precancerous lesions and to investigate the pathogenesis of the disease. HPV plays a major role in the development of cervical cancer, but histological types have different relationships with HPV genotypes. HPV can remain latent for a long time and the most important thing determining the persistence is the type of HPV. HPV vaccination provides a direct benefit to both men and women by providing safe protection against cancers that may result from persistent HPV infection.

Keywords: cervical cancer, human papillomavirus, casualty, etiology, screening, vaccine

1. Introduction

Worldwide, cervical cancer is the fourth most common cancer among females and the third most common female genital tract cancer. 570,000 cases of invasive cervical carcinoma were diagnosed and 311,000 cervical cancer deaths occurred in 2018 [1, 2]. In low-income countries that do not have access to cervical cancer screening and prevention programs, cervical cancer continues to be a major cause of cancer diseases and deaths. The prevalence of cervical cancer and precancerous lesions depends on how effectively cancer screening programs and HPV vaccines are used in populations. The causal relationship between HPV and cervical cancer has been well documented [3–6] and HPV can be detected in 99.7 percent of cervical cancers [7]. Studies have consistently shown strong geographical correlations between HPV-DNA prevalence and cervical cancer incidence [6]. The worldwide spot prevalence of HPV is about 10 percent detected in a meta-analysis of studies involving more than 150,000 images with normal cervical cytology [8].

Africa is the most prevalent place of HPV infection in the world, where HPV is detected in 22% of African women. The most common types worldwide are HPV types 16 and 18, however, there appears to be geographic variation in the distribution of HPV genotypes.

HPV causes oropharyngeal and anogenital diseases in both men and women and is usually sexually transmitted. HPV infections are considered the most common sexually transmitted disease in sexually active individuals. It is estimated that at least 80% of sexually active individuals have been exposed to HPV once in their lifetime [9].

The most common histological type of cervical cancer is squamous cell carcinoma (SCC) (70%). Although the incidence of invasive cervical adenocarcinoma and its variants has gradually increased in the last few years; this type of neoplasia accounts for approximately 25% of all invasive cervical cancers diagnosed today. Other rare variants also constitute 3–5% of cervical cancer. HPV plays a major role in the development of cervical cancer, but histological types have different relationships with HPV genotypes. Available data state that HPV 18 accounts for 15% of SCCs and about 50% of adenocarcinomas [10]. The highest prevalence of HPV infection typically occurs within the first decade after sexual intercourse, typically between the ages of 15 and 25 in most western countries. Many sexually active young women have sequential infections with different types of oncogenic HPV. These infections are usually detected temporarily, but often reversible cytological changes occur. HPV spreads from the skin to the skin surface, and cutaneous HPV infections are common in the general population. Person-to-person transitions are typically asymptomatic [11]. Therefore, unprotected penetrative sexual intercourse (both vaginal and anal) or close physical contact from skin to skin is the most important factor for HPV infection [12]. Other risk factors are the number of partners [13, 14], new sexual partners [14], high-risk sexual partner, previous sexually transmitted disease, young age, not being married, non-Hispanic black, being the highest school graduate, poverty, low-income, first coitus at younger than 18 years old [8], primary or secondary immunodeficiency conditions. Spread from other HPV-infected genital organs, such as post-toilet wiping from front to back, may also play a role in the transmission of other types of contact [14, 15]. Penetrating vaginal and anal intercourse is not required for passage, but the prevalence of infection is much lower in virgins. Female-to-male transmission may occur at a higher rate than male-to-female transmission [16]. Regular condom use reduces the risk of HPV infection [17]. However, condoms do not completely prevent the transmission of HPV because the virus is spread through skin-to-skin contact.

HPV usually makes its first peak at an early age in unvaccinated sexually active women. Humoral and cellular immunity is provided with natural immunity partially [18, 19]. The presence of anti-HPV antibodies in patients with previous HPV type 16 infection has been associated with a lower risk of infection later, and it is thought that protective immunity is formed [18, 20–22]. However, it is not known how long and how much this protection lasts. It has been documented that some individuals with HPV infection did not develop antibodies [22, 23]. The second peak is in the postmenopausal period [24, 25]. This may be due to weakened cellular immunity or persistence or reactivation of a previously acquired infection. Reactivation may be the main source of newly detected HPV infection in HIV-positive women [26]. The oncogenic activity of HPV increases in the postmenopausal period. New HPV infection in older women does not usually progress to preinvasive disease or cancer.

HPV can remain latent for a long time and the most important thing determining the persistence is the type of HPV. HPV infection is best documented by molecular tests. PCR and in situ hybridization are mostly used in HPV typing.

With cytological examinations, only 30% of the patients represent the presence of a cytological disorder caused by HPV. A high-risk HPV type is responsible for 95% of pre-invasive lesions of the cervix and cervical cancer.

HPV has more than 200 types and can be divided into subgroups as mucous or cutaneous types according to their tissue tropism. Typing depends on DNA sequence and homology. Each type was separately identified as having less than 90% DNA base pair homology with another HPV strain. In addition to HPV genotypes, HPV intratypic variants also have epidemiological and oncogenic value in cervical cancer [27]. Different HPV types tend to infect different parts of the human body and are therefore associated with different diseases. The most common types of HPV associated with certain lesions vary according to the geography and demography of the population studied, but generally HPV types 6 and 11 cause condyloma acuminata, while type 16,18,31,52 cause intraepithelial neoplasms of the cervix [26, 28]. Over 40 HPV types showing tropism to the anogenital epithelium enter the epithelium of the penis, scrotum, perineum, anal canal, perianal area, vaginal introitus, vulva, and cervix. Approximately 15 HPV types are known as high risk, carcinogenic, or cancer-related [8]. High risk HPV types; 16, 18, 31, 33, 35, 39, 45, 51, 52, 56, 58, 59, and 68 low-risk HPV types; 6, 11, 40, 42, 43, 44, 53, 54, 61, 72, 73, and 8. Among these, the most common HPV type in cervical cancer is type 16, and the intraepithelial neoplasia it causes is the type most likely to progress to cancer [3]. The reason of low-risk HPV types not causing cancer is that they cannot integrate into the host cell's chromosome. The E6 and E7 genes of such HPV viruses bind weakly to p53 and pRb. The presence of a cervical transformation site is not necessary for oncogenic HPV to infect the female genital tract. Because HPV can also cause cancer in the vulva, vagina, and anal region, the epithelium of which is mentioned before, squamous keratinized epithelium. HPV 18 causes disease more frequently in younger women and recurrence is more than that of HPV 16. In cervical cancer, the specificity of HPV 18 is higher than that of HPV 16. HPV 16 and 18 involve the cervix more than other HPV types with low oncogenic potential.

2. Basic virology

The link between genital HPV infections and cervical cancer was first demonstrated in the early1980s by Harold Zur Hausen, since then, the biology of HPV viruses has been extensively studied and has proven well connected with neoplasia.

HPV is an epithelotrophic virus from the Papillomaviridae family, small, non-enveloped, encapsulated, 55 nm in diameter, containing double helix 8 kilobase circular DNA. Human papillomaviruses are a big family with the systematic classification of five genera (α, β, γ, μ, and ν), 48 species, and 206 types [27]. The genetic map of HPV-16 is illustrated in **Figure 1** [29]. It is coated with 72-surface icosahedral protein capsid which contains at least two capsid proteins, L1 and L2. HPV genome contains 7900 base pairs. It encodes 8 genes that can encode early and late proteins and URR, which control the transcription of late genes without coding [30]. Early proteins are associated with viral gene regulation and cell transformation, while late proteins form the coat of the virus [31, 32]. Specific gene products are duplicated at each differentiation level of squamous keratinocyte [33]. At the most superficial level, the L1, L2, and E4 genes are duplicated for assembly of the viral capsid in which the HPV genome is packaged. After the short-lived superficial cells desquamate, infectious HPV virions are released for the next round of infection. E1,2,5,6 and 7 are expressed in the early period of differentiation of HPV in the epithelium, L1 and L2 are expressed in the late period, and E4 is expressed during differentiation. E4 is the gene most associated with viral release. E1 and E2 play

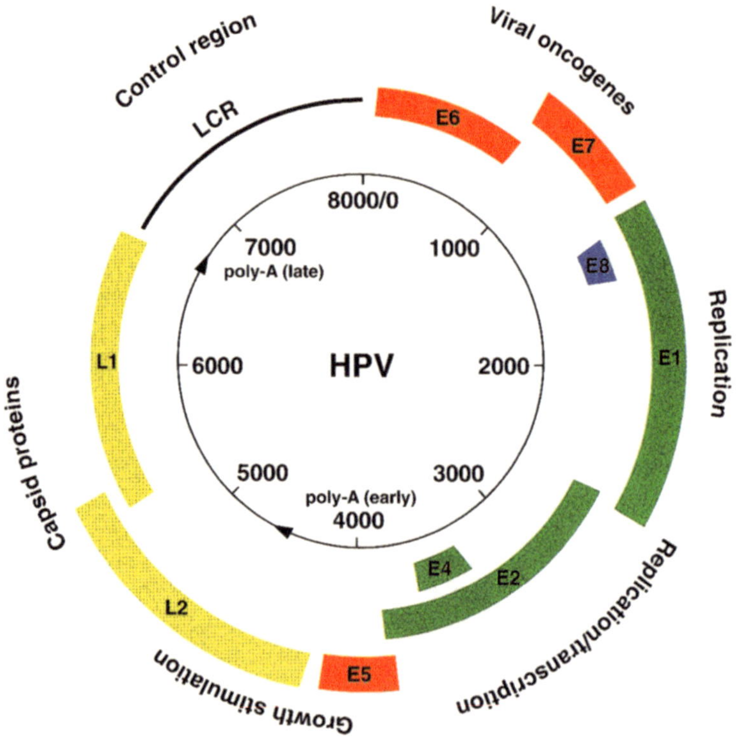

Figure 1.
Genome organization of human papillomavirus. The genetic map of HPV-16.

a critical role in participating in the structure of host DNA. E1 enables the regulation of DNA replication and keeping the virus in episomal form. E2 cooperates with E1, ensures viral DNA replication, downregulates E6 and E7 expression [34]. The HPV genome remains a stable viral episome in the nucleus of the cell, independent of the host cell nucleus. When it causes cervical cancer or pre-invasive diseases of the cervix, the HPV genome in the host nucleus integrates into the host cell's DNA. Viral integration into cellular DNA was proposed as a marker of progression to cervical cancer. Integration is rarely seen in the pre-invasive disease. Whether integration in HSIL stages progresses to cervical cancer is unknown [6]. When E2 is added to the DNA structure, it degrades and as a result, E6 and E7 expression is increased [35]. In other words, the production of E6 and E7 is mainly under the control of E2. E6 and E7 are the major HPV oncoproteins and they work together to immortalize epithelial cells [36]. Both E6 and E7 proteins are consistently expressed in cancerous tissues. E6 can lead to persistent infections and invasive cancer development with its telomerase activity. E6 activates c-myc and increases telomerase activity of the catalytic subunit gene (by increasing hTERT transcription) [37]. It has also been shown that E6 and E7 antagonize the inhibition of hTERT via BRCA [38].

E6 and E7 proteins of HPV 16 bind more tightly to their targets than other HPV types, so HPV 16 becomes more persistent. E6 binds and suppresses p53, which blocks the G1 → S step in the cell cycle [39]. Following E6 binding of p53, p53 is disrupted in the presence of E6-associated protein [40]. If p53 does not participate, DNA damage cannot be repaired. The result is that the global cycle cannot be controlled, there is no apoptosis, and chromosomal mutations accumulate because there is no DNA repair [41, 42]. E7 binds to the retinoblastoma that regulates apoptosis and forces the cell to enter the synthesis step [33]. Retinablostome inactivates the E2F transcription factor that controls DNA synthesis, cyclin function and promotes the S phase of the cell cycle. When E7 binds to the Rb protein, E2F is released, allowing cyclin A to promote cell turnover [43]. Thus, a cell with unstable chromosomes and high-risk HPV can turn into a malignant cell. E6 and E7 are essential proteins in immortality transformation. But these two genes are not the only ones responsible for cancer development [44]. Progression to neoplasia possibly involves a genetic change in the pathways that control intracellular or intercellular signaling [45].

E5, on the other hand, disrupts the antigen presentation of MHC-I and MHC-II. E5 also activates the EGF pathway [34]. The L1 protein self-assembles in the absence of the viral genome to form a virus-like particle (VLP). L1 VLP is the immunogen used in HPV vaccines. L2 is the minor capsid protein that mediates HPV infection with L1 [46, 47].

3. HPV infection causality in cervical cancer

The role of the HPV virus in cervical cancer development is proven by the demonstration of HPV DNA and viral oncogenes E6 and E7 in cancerous tissues, that E6 and E7 gene products have host cell transforming properties, and HPV has been shown as a major factor in cervical cancer development in epidemiological studies. There are four main steps in the development of cervical cancer [48];

1. One or more oncogenic types of HPV infection of the metaplastic epithelium at the cervical transformation zone,

2. Persistence of the HPV infection rather than clearance,

3. Progression of a clone of epithelial cells from persistent viral infection to precancer (CIN3)

4. Carcinoma invasion through the basement membrane

Initial infection of the basal cell of cervical epithelium occurs as a result of microscopic breaks in the epithelium [33]. HPV targets and binds to the heparin sulfate proteoglycan receptor located in the basement membrane [49] indicating that HPV infection starts from the basement membrane. The replication cycle of the virus depends on the maturation of the keratinocyte. Since HPV does not enter the bloodstream, it does not cause viremia and inflammation. Therefore, the antigen is not formed against HPV and HPV cannot be detected by blood tests. There are also no FDA-approved serological or blood tests to detect HPV infection.

Although HPV infection is common in the population, cervical cancer develops in a minority of these infected patients. Because most HPV infections are temporary and additional factors are required for cancer development. The period from the first infection with HPV to the development of cancer is approximately 15 years. Different subtypes of HPV are detected at different rates in histological types of cervical cancer. In squamous cell carcinoma, HPV 16,18,58,33and 45 is found in 59%, 13%, 5%,5% and 4% of cases,respectively. In adenocarcinoma, HPV 16,18,45,31 and 33 is found in 36%, 37%, 5% percent, 2%,2% of cases, respectively [2].

The most expected and most likely outcome in women infected with HPV is complete resolution of the infection within 2 years [50, 51]. The least expected result is the development of neoplasia [52] and it occurs as a result of persistent infection. Currently, there is no effective treatment for HPV persistence [53].

Spontaneous recovery of HPV infection is more likely in young women [6]. Low-grade lesions caused by HPV can be detected clinically when smears are used for screening, but they are usually temporary, however, HPV can become latent [54]. It may be reactivated in immunocompromised patients however, it is not known which HPV infections become latent and whether recurrent HPV infections carry a significant cancer risk. The possibility of pre-cancerous or cancerous lesions increases with persistent HPV infections. More than one HPV type can be positive in a woman. When women with multiple types of infection were compared with women who were positive for only one HPV type, no increased risk was identified. This suggests that each HPV type causes disease independently from the other [55].

Although HPV is the most powerful cause for cervical cancer development, the presence of HPV alone is not sufficient for cervical cancer, and additional factors are required. These factors can be causes such as smoking, endogenous and exogenous hormones. HPV is positive in 99% of patients diagnosed with cervical cancer. It is thought that an HPV virus type that causes cervical cancer is encountered around the age of 21 on average [56]. While HPV 16 is responsible for 50% of cervical cancer, HPV 18 is responsible for 20% [57]. The remaining cases (19%) are caused by HPV 31,33,45,52,58 [58]. While persistent HPV infection progressing to CIN3 in 5 years [59], CIN3 progresses to invasive cancer in 30% of patients after 30 years [60]. Factors such as smoking, multiparity, age at first birth, and the use of oral contraceptives facilitate the progression of HPV-infected epithelial cells to cancer [61].

Excessive viral load in the lesion does not mean that the lesion will progress to cancer, except for HPV 16 [62]. Very high dose viral load may be detected in some low-grade lesions, but these lesions may regress over time [8]. Therefore, viral load measurement is not useful in the clinic and does not provide any additional benefit [63].

4. HPV vaccination

Routine HPV vaccination is recommended for adolescents and young adults in many countries. HPV vaccination provides a direct benefit to both men and women by providing safe protection against cancers that may result from persistent HPV infection. This protective effect has been best demonstrated in cervical cancer, one of the most common women's cancers worldwide. Inactive HPV vaccination can prevent HPV infection and its sequelae. Vaccination status does not change recommendations for screening. HPV vaccine provides protection not only from cervical caser but also from vulvar, vaginal, oropharyngeal, anal cancers, and anogenital warts. There is also evidence of decreased genital warts among men of similar age in areas with a high proportion of vaccinated women [64].

The vaccine does not protect against 100 percent of the types known to cause cervical cancer since the most extensive vaccine protects against only 9 types of HPV. Therefore, women should continue to have cervical screening regardless of whether they are vaccinated or not. However, in societies that cannot include the HPV vaccine in the routine vaccination program due to economic concerns, it is recommended that public health efforts focus primarily on the vaccination of young women, the group with the absolute benefit and cost-effectiveness of HPV vaccination. However, none of the existing HPV vaccines will cure pre-existing vaccine-type HPV infections or related diseases [27], as the vaccine is effective if used in primary prevention. Sexually active individuals should be vaccinated consistently with recommendations specific to their age. Abnormal Papanicolaou test, genital warts, or a history of HPV infection is not a contraindication to HPV vaccination [65]. The HPV vaccine is recommended for these patients as it can still protect against infection with HPV vaccine types that have not been encountered yet [66, 67]. However, if the individual is previously infected with any HPV type in the vaccine, it reduces the protection of the vaccine.

These vaccines contain virus-like particles, but without producing the effect of the virus, only activate the body's immune system, in other words, by initiating the production of HPV-type antibodies, enable the woman to become resistant to HPV for a long time. Many studies have reported that the prevalence and incidence of HPV infection and HPV-related disease decreased following the initiation of HPV vaccination [68–71].

The vaccine does not contain virus DNA, it contains capsid particles of the virus. The vaccine is produced against the L1 and L2 capsid proteins. L1 VLP vaccines strongly stimulate cellular and humoral immunity. There are three types of HPV vaccine, bivalent, quadrivalent, and 9-in-1 vaccine, although not all of them are available everywhere. Bivalent vaccine is protective against the HPV types 16 and 18, quadrivalent vaccine and 9-shot to vaccine to,HPV types 16,18,6,11, and HPV types 16,18,6,11,31,33,45,52,58 respectively. Although it is not available everywhere, it is more advantageous to be vaccinated with a 9-shot vaccine since it contains more HPV types that cause cervical cancer. Characteristics of the three human papillomaviruses (HPV) vaccines licensed for use in the United States are demonstrated in **Table 1** [72]. Therapeutic vaccines are under development but not clinically available [73].

The best time for HPV vaccination is before an individual has sexual intercourse. Clinical trial data on vaccine efficacy in men and women show that vaccination with the HPV vaccine is most effective among people not infected with HPV. Although it can be applied to individuals of all age groups, routine HPV vaccination is recommended between 11 and 12 years of age [66]. In this age group, the protection of the vaccine is almost 100% [74–77]. The resulting titers are generally higher in younger people than in older individuals [72]. There is no minimum threshold titer defined for protection. The natural history and the determinants of the immune response to HPV are still poorly understood [6]. The World Health Organization (WHO)

Characteristic	Bivalent (2vHPV)	Quadrivalent (4vHPV)	9-valent (9vHPV)
Brand name	Cervarix	Gardasil	Gardasil 9
VLPs	16, 18	6,11,16,18	6, 11, 16, 18, 31, 33, 45, 52, 58
Manufacturer	GlaxoSmithKline	Merck and Co., Inc	Merck and Co., Inc
Manufacturing	*Trichoplusia ni* insect cell line infected with L1 encoding recombinant baculovirus	*Saccharomyces cerevisiae* (Baker's yeast), expressing L1	Saccharomyces cerevisiae (Baker's yeast), expressing L1
Adjuvant	500 μg aluminum hydroxide, 50 μg 3-O-desacyl-4′ monophosphoryl lipid A	225 μg amorphous aluminum hydroxyphosphate sulfate	500 μg amorphous aluminum hydroxyphosphate sulfate
Volume per dose	0.5 ml	0.5 ml	0.5 ml
Administration	Intramuscular	Intramuscular	Intramuscular

Table 1.
Characteristics of the three human papillomavirus (HPV) vaccines licensed for use in the United States.

recommends that the primary target of HPV vaccination programs is women between the ages of 9 and 14 and that local public health programs only recommend that older women be vaccinated if it is cost-effective and does not divert resources from vaccinating the primary target population or cervical cancer screening [66]. It is recommended to vaccinate men between the ages of 16–26 [72]. The vaccine can be administered from the age of 9 years [72], but it is not recommended before the age of 9. Compensatory vaccination is recommended for adolescents and adults aged 13–26 who have not been vaccinated before or have not completed the vaccine series [78] and for males aged 13 through 21 years who have not been vaccinated previously or who have not completed the 3-dose series. Males aged 22 through 26 years may be vaccinated. ACIP recommends vaccination of men who have sex with men and immunocompromised persons through age 26 years if not vaccinated previously [72]. The decision to vaccinate individuals over the age of 26 should be made on an individual basis. Because in this age group, the protection of the vaccine decreases [79]. While the protection of the vaccine is 81% in individuals between the ages of 26–35, it decreases to 75% in individuals between the ages of 35–46. The rate of protection is 44% in individuals who have been previously infected with HPV [80]. In these cases, the vaccine protects against other types of HPV. Persons who are virgin under the age of 26 can have the 9-inoculation vaccine if they have had a bivalent or quadrivalent vaccine before. The HPV vaccine is not recommended during pregnancy due to limited safety information [72]. Those who were vaccinated by mistake during pregnancy do not need termination because no relationship has been shown between the HPV vaccine and abortion or poor fetal outcomes [81]. Women of reproductive age do not need a pregnancy test before vaccination [72]. If conception is achieved between doses, the remaining doses are postponed, the remaining doses are completed after pregnancy, and do not start over [82]. Vaccine is safe for nursing mothers because inactive vaccines do not affect the safety of breastfeeding. There is no need to screen the individual for HPV before HPV vaccination [67]. Measurement of post-vaccination antibody titers has no clinical use [6] since the protective titer is unknown.

In addition, studies are showing that HPV is present in the smoke that occurs during the surgical removal or ablation of HPV-infected tissues and that nasal or oropharyngeal HPV infection may develop if this smoke is inhaled by healthcare workers [83]. Therefore, it would be beneficial to vaccinate healthcare workers who are at risk of such exposure [84]. Studies have shown that the HPV vaccine protects women against high-grade lesions of the cervix, vulva, and vagina for 10 years, and persistent antibody levels have been found [85–87].

The vaccine is administered in 3 doses [72]. The peak immunity achieved with 3 doses of vaccination is greater than that of native HPV infection. After 2 years, the antibody level drops but is still higher than that of innate immunity [78]. There is no evidence of the additional benefit of a booster dose. For individuals under 15 years of age, 2 doses are sufficient (between 0 and 6–12 months). In this age group, if the second dose is administered less than five months after the first dose, the dose should be repeated at least 12 weeks after the second dose and at least five months after the first dose. It can be applied in 0,1 and 6 months or 0, 2, and 6 months. The interval between the first and second doses should be a minimum of 4 weeks. The interval between the second and third doses should be a minimum of 12 weeks. The minimum interval between the first and third doses should be 5 months. If a dose has been administered at a shorter interval, it should be repeated at the minimum recommended interval after the last dose has passed [66, 67, 88]. If the dosing schedule is got out of order the remaining doses are made quickly, not starting over [67, 72]. Vaccines that can provide the same protection after 1 dose are in the development phase. Such a vaccine could be an important breakthrough for low-income countries to prevent disease. If possible, the vaccination should be continued with whatever type of vaccine it started. However, if there is a problem in accessing the vaccine or if the first vaccine is not known, it can be continued with other types of vaccines [72]. Although direct efficacy data on HPV vaccination in immunocompromised hosts are lacking, immunocompromised individuals can also be vaccinated in the same manner [66]. The HPV vaccine can be safely administered in a different anatomical region at the same time with other age-appropriate vaccines. Coadministration of HPV vaccine with other vaccines does not affect the immune response [83, 89].

Side effects of HPV vaccination are generally limited to mild local reactions (regional reaction, systemic malaise, fever) [72] and syncope. Mild injection site reactions were the most common side effects in studies [90]. Syncope is not specific to the HPV vaccine [90, 91]. None of the side effects already seen are characteristic of the HPV vaccine. Following HPV vaccination, a routine waiting period of 15 minutes in a sitting or supine position is recommended [67]. Other reported side effects include headache, nausea, vomiting, tiredness, dizziness, and weakness [43]. The adjuvant aluminum hydroxyphosphate found in the quadrivalent and 9-vaccine and the adjuvant aluminum hydroxide + monophosphoryl lipid found in the bivalent vaccine is used to increase the immunological response of the vaccine. The higher the amount of adjuvant in the vaccine, the more side effects it has. For this reason, since the 9-vaccine contains more adjuvant substances, its side effects occur more [72]. However, the protection of the 9-in-1 vaccine against HPV 16 and 18 is approximately as much as the quadrivalent vaccine [72].

5. Conclusions

Cervical cancer is preventable cancer worldwide with the organized and strict compliance of early screening methods, vaccination programs, and changing sexual behavior. Aggressive treatments of early or ambiguous cytologic lesions related to HPV may result in a decrease in rates of more advanced disease although increases in the incidence of cervical adenocarcinomas have been reported in several populations. Because cervical screening tests are insufficient in detecting adenocarcinoma. Since the HPV vaccine is protective against high-risk types, it is beneficial to apply it to the recommended age groups.

Acknowledgements

Thank you very much to Ömer Harun Sağnıç,M.D. and Özer Birge,M.D. for their contributions and supports.

No financial support has been received in writing this article.

Conflict of interest

The author declare no conflict of interest.

Notes/thanks/other declarations

None.

Author details

Saliha Sağnıç
Division of Gynecologic Oncology, Department of Gynecology Obstetrics, Akdeniz University, Antalya, Turkey

*Address all correspondence to: drsalihasagnic@hotmail.com

References

[1] Arbyn, M., et al., Estimates of incidence and mortality of cervical cancer in 2018: a worldwide analysis. Lancet Glob Health, 2020. 8(2): p. e191-e203.

[2] Siegel, R.L., et al., Cancer Statistics, 2021. CA Cancer J Clin, 2021. 71(1): p. 7-33.

[3] Franco, E.L., E. Duarte-Franco, and A. Ferenczy, Cervical cancer: epidemiology, prevention and the role of human papillomavirus infection. Cmaj, 2001. 164(7): p. 1017-25.

[4] Sedlacek, T.V., Advances in the diagnosis and treatment of human papillomavirus infections. Clin Obstet Gynecol, 1999. 42(2): p. 206-20.

[5] Sonnex, C., Human papillomavirus infection with particular reference to genital disease. J Clin Pathol, 1998. 51(9): p. 643-8.

[6] Lei, J., et al., HPV Vaccination and the Risk of Invasive Cervical Cancer. N Engl J Med, 2020. 383(14): p. 1340-1348.

[7] Comparison of risk factors for invasive squamous cell carcinoma and adenocarcinoma of the cervix: collaborative reanalysis of individual data on 8,097 women with squamous cell carcinoma and 1,374 women with adenocarcinoma from 12 epidemio logical studies. Int J Cancer, 2007. 120(4): p. 885-91.

[8] Schiffman, M., et al., Human papillomavirus and cervical cancer. Lancet, 2007. 370(9590): p. 890-907.

[9] Brotherton, J.M., et al., Early effect of the HPV vaccination programme on cervical abnormalities in Victoria, Australia: an ecological study. Lancet, 2011. 377(9783): p. 2085-92.

[10] Oshman, L.D. and A.M. Davis, Human Papillomavirus Vaccination for Adults: Updated Recommendations of the Advisory Committee on Immunization Practices (ACIP). Jama, 2020. 323(5): p. 468-469.

[11] Castellsagué, X., et al., Risk of newly detected infections and cervical abnormalities in women seropositive for naturally acquired human papillomavirus type 16/18 antibodies: analysis of the control arm of PATRICIA. J Infect Dis, 2014. 210(4): p. 517-34.

[12] Tarkowski, T.A., et al., Epidemiology of human papillomavirus infection and abnormal cytologic test results in an urban adolescent population. J Infect Dis, 2004. 189(1): p. 46-50.

[13] Winer, R.L., et al., Genital human papillomavirus infection: incidence and risk factors in a cohort of female university students. Am J Epidemiol, 2003. 157(3): p. 218-26.

[14] Simpson, S., Jr., et al., Front-to-back & dabbing wiping behaviour post-toilet associated with anal neoplasia & HR-HPV carriage in women with previous HPV-mediated gynaecological neoplasia. Cancer Epidemiol, 2016. 42: p. 124-32.

[15] Nyitray, A.G., et al., The role of monogamy and duration of heterosexual relationships in human papillomavirus transmission. J Infect Dis, 2014. 209(7): p. 1007-15.

[16] Dunne, E.F., et al., Prevalence of HPV infection among men: A systematic review of the literature. J Infect Dis, 2006. 194(8): p. 1044-57.

[17] Trimble, C.L., et al., Safety, efficacy, and immunogenicity of VGX-3100, a therapeutic synthetic DNA vaccine targeting human papillomavirus 16 and 18 E6 and E7 proteins for cervical

intraepithelial neoplasia 2/3: a randomised, double-blind, placebo-controlled phase 2b trial. Lancet, 2015. 386(10008): p. 2078-2088.

[18] Safaeian, M., et al., Epidemiological study of anti-HPV16/18 seropositivity and subsequent risk of HPV16 and –18 infections. J Natl Cancer Inst, 2010. 102(21): p. 1653-62.

[19] Lehtinen, M., et al., Overall efficacy of HPV-16/18 AS04-adjuvanted vaccine against grade 3 or greater cervical intraepithelial neoplasia: 4-year end-of-study analysis of the randomised, double-blind PATRICIA trial. Lancet Oncol, 2012. 13(1): p. 89-99.

[20] Wilson, L., et al., Seroprevalence of 8 oncogenic human papillomavirus genotypes and acquired immunity against reinfection. J Infect Dis, 2014. 210(3): p. 448-55.

[21] Safaeian, M., et al., Risk of HPV-16/18 Infections and Associated Cervical Abnormalities in Women Seropositive for Naturally Acquired Antibodies: Pooled Analysis Based on Control Arms of Two Large Clinical Trials. J Infect Dis, 2018. 218(1): p. 84-94.

[22] Wentzensen, N., et al., A competitive serological assay shows naturally acquired immunity to human papillomavirus infections in the Guanacaste Natural History Study. J Infect Dis, 2011. 204(1): p. 94-102.

[23] Winer, R.L., et al., Condom use and the risk of genital human papillomavirus infection in young women. N Engl J Med, 2006. 354(25): p. 2645-54.

[24] Herrero, R., et al., Epidemiologic profile of type-specific human papillomavirus infection and cervical neoplasia in Guanacaste, Costa Rica. J Infect Dis, 2005. 191(11): p. 1796-807.

[25] Strickler, H.D., et al., Natural history and possible reactivation of human papillomavirus in human immunodeficiency virus-positive women. J Natl Cancer Inst, 2005. 97(8): p. 577-86.

[26] Burchell, A.N., et al., Chapter 6: Epidemiology and transmission dynamics of genital HPV infection. Vaccine, 2006. 24 Suppl 3: p. S3/52-61.

[27] Hu, Z. and D. Ma, The precision prevention and therapy of HPV-related cervical cancer: new concepts and clinical implications. Cancer Med, 2018. 7(10): p. 5217-5236.

[28] Insinga, R.P., et al., A systematic review of the prevalence and attribution of human papillomavirus types among cervical, vaginal, and vulvar precancers and cancers in the United States. Cancer Epidemiol Biomarkers Prev, 2008. 17(7): p. 1611-22.

[29] Antonishyn, N., The utility of hpv typing and relative quantification of HPV-16 transcripts for monitoring HPV vaccine efficacy and improving colposcopy triage of women with abnormal cervical cytology. 2021.

[30] Klingelhutz, A.J., S.A. Foster, and J.K. McDougall, Telomerase activation by the E6 gene product of human papillomavirus type 16. Nature, 1996. 380(6569): p. 79-82.

[31] Palefsky, J.M., Anal human papillomavirus infection and anal cancer in HIV-positive individuals: an emerging problem. Aids, 1994. 8(3): p. 283-95.

[32] Münger, K., et al., The E6 and E7 genes of the human papillomavirus type 16 together are necessary and sufficient for transformation of primary human keratinocytes. J Virol, 1989. 63(10): p. 4417-21.

[33] Doorbar, J., Molecular biology of human papillomavirus infection and

cervical cancer. Clin Sci (Lond), 2006. 110(5): p. 525-41.

[34] Schwarz, E., et al., Structure and transcription of human papillomavirus sequences in cervical carcinoma cells. Nature, 1985. 314(6006): p. 111-4.

[35] zur Hausen, H., Papillomaviruses causing cancer: evasion from host-cell control in early events in carcinogenesis. J Natl Cancer Inst, 2000. 92(9): p. 690-8.

[36] Scheffner, M., et al., The HPV-16 E6 and E6-AP complex functions as a ubiquitin-protein ligase in the ubiquitination of p53. Cell, 1993. 75(3): p. 495-505.

[37] Scheffner, M., et al., The E6 oncoprotein encoded by human papillomavirus types 16 and 18 promotes the degradation of p53. Cell, 1990. 63(6): p. 1129-36.

[38] Dyson, N., et al., The human papilloma virus-16 E7 oncoprotein is able to bind to the retinoblastoma gene product. Science, 1989. 243(4893): p. 934-7.

[39] zur Hausen, H., Papillomaviruses and cancer: from basic studies to clinical application. Nat Rev Cancer, 2002. 2(5): p. 342-50.

[40] Havre, P.A., et al., p53 inactivation by HPV16 E6 results in increased mutagenesis in human cells. Cancer Res, 1995. 55(19): p. 4420-4.

[41] Werness, B.A., A.J. Levine, and P.M. Howley, Association of human papillomavirus types 16 and 18 E6 proteins with p53. Science, 1990. 248(4951): p. 76-9.

[42] Puthenveettil, J.A., S.M. Frederickson, and C.A. Reznikoff, Apoptosis in human papillomavirus16 E7-, but not E6-immortalized human uroepithelial cells. Oncogene, 1996. 13(6): p. 1123-31.

[43] Palefsky, J.M. and E.A. Holly, Molecular virology and epidemiology of human papillomavirus and cervical cancer. Cancer Epidemiol Biomarkers Prev, 1995. 4(4): p. 415-28.

[44] Burger, E.A., et al., Age of Acquiring Causal Human Papillomavirus (HPV) Infections: Leveraging Simulation Models to Explore the Natural History of HPV-induced Cervical Cancer. Clin Infect Dis, 2017. 65(6): p. 893-899.

[45] Schiffman, M., et al., Human papillomavirus testing in the prevention of cervical cancer. J Natl Cancer Inst, 2011. 103(5): p. 368-83.

[46] Yang, R., et al., Interaction of L2 with beta-actin directs intracellular transport of papillomavirus and infection. J Biol Chem, 2003. 278(14): p. 12546-53.

[47] Yang, R., et al., Cell surface-binding motifs of L2 that facilitate papillomavirus infection. J Virol, 2003. 77(6): p. 3531-41.

[48] Li, N., et al., Human papillomavirus type distribution in 30,848 invasive cervical cancers worldwide: Variation by geographical region, histological type and year of publication. Int J Cancer, 2011. 128(4): p. 927-35.

[49] Johnson, K.M., et al., Role of heparan sulfate in attachment to and infection of the murine female genital tract by human papillomavirus. J Virol, 2009. 83(5): p. 2067-74.

[50] Stanley, M., Immune responses to human papillomavirus. Vaccine, 2006. 24 Suppl 1: p. S16-22.

[51] Plummer, M., et al., A 2-year prospective study of human papillomavirus persistence among

women with a cytological diagnosis of atypical squamous cells of undetermined significance or low-grade squamous intraepithelial lesion. J Infect Dis, 2007. 195(11): p. 1582-9.

[52] Woodman, C.B., S.I. Collins, and L.S. Young, The natural history of cervical HPV infection: unresolved issues. Nat Rev Cancer, 2007. 7(1): p. 11-22.

[53] Hu, Z., et al., TALEN-mediated targeting of HPV oncogenes ameliorates HPV-related cervical malignancy. J Clin Invest, 2015. 125(1): p. 425-36.

[54] Maglennon, G.A. and J. Doorbar, The biology of papillomavirus latency. Open Virol J, 2012. 6: p. 190-7.

[55] Muñoz, N., et al., Epidemiologic classification of human papillomavirus types associated with cervical cancer. N Engl J Med, 2003. 348(6): p. 518-27.

[56] Ylitalo, N., et al., Consistent high viral load of human papillomavirus 16 and risk of cervical carcinoma in situ: a nested case-control study. Lancet, 2000. 355(9222): p. 2194-8.

[57] Serrano, B., et al. Potential impact of a nine-valent vaccine in human papillomavirus related cervical disease. Infect Agent Cancer 2012 Dec 29 [cited 7 1]; 2013/01/01:[38].

[58] Available from: https://www.cdc.gov/std/hpv/stdfact-hpv.htm.

[59] McCredie, M.R., et al., Natural history of cervical neoplasia and risk of invasive cancer in women with cervical intraepithelial neoplasia 3: a retrospective cohort study. Lancet Oncol, 2008. 9(5): p. 425-34.

[60] Appleby, P., et al., Carcinoma of the cervix and tobacco smoking: collaborative reanalysis of individual data on 13,541 women with carcinoma of the cervix and 23,017 women without carcinoma of the cervix from 23 epidemiological studies. Int J Cancer, 2006. 118(6): p. 1481-95.

[61] Van Tine, B.A., et al., Human papillomavirus (HPV) origin-binding protein associates with mitotic spindles to enable viral DNA partitioning. Proc Natl Acad Sci U S A, 2004. 101(12): p. 4030-5.

[62] Sherman, M.E., et al., Determinants of human papillomavirus load among women with histological cervical intraepithelial neoplasia 3: dominant impact of surrounding low-grade lesions. Cancer Epidemiol Biomarkers Prev, 2003. 12(10): p. 1038-44.

[63] Bosch, F.X. and S. de Sanjosé, Chapter 1: Human papillomavirus and cervical cancer--burden and assessment of causality. J Natl Cancer Inst Monogr, 2003(31): p. 3-13.

[64] Hughes, J.P., G.P. Garnett, and L. Koutsky, The theoretical population-level impact of a prophylactic human papilloma virus vaccine. Epidemiology, 2002. 13(6): p. 631-9.

[65] Freedman, M., et al., Recommended Adult Immunization Schedule, United States, 2020. Ann Intern Med, 2020. 172(5): p. 337-347.

[66] Markowitz, L.E., et al., Human papillomavirus vaccination: recommendations of the Advisory Committee on Immunization Practices (ACIP). MMWR Recomm Rep, 2014. 63(Rr-05): p. 1-30.

[67] Robinson, C.L., et al., Advisory Committee on Immunization Practices Recommended Immunization Schedule for Children and Adolescents Aged 18 Years or Younger - United States, 2020. MMWR Morb Mortal Wkly Rep, 2020. 69(5): p. 130-132.

[68] Tabrizi, S.N., et al., Fall in human papillomavirus prevalence following a

national vaccination program. J Infect Dis, 2012. 206(11): p. 1645-51.

[69] Donovan, B., et al., Quadrivalent human papillomavirus vaccination and trends in genital warts in Australia: analysis of national sentinel surveillance data. Lancet Infect Dis, 2011. 11(1): p. 39-44.

[70] Berenson, A.B., T.H. Laz, and M. Rahman, Reduction in Vaccine-Type Human Papillomavirus Prevalence Among Women in the United States, 2009-2012. J Infect Dis, 2016. 214(12): p. 1961-1964.

[71] de Sanjosé, S., et al., Worldwide prevalence and genotype distribution of cervical human papillomavirus DNA in women with normal cytology: a meta-analysis. Lancet Infect Dis, 2007. 7(7): p. 453-9.

[72] Petrosky, E., et al., Use of 9-valent human papillomavirus (HPV) vaccine: updated HPV vaccination recommendations of the advisory committee on immunization practices. MMWR Morb Mortal Wkly Rep, 2015. 64(11): p. 300-4.

[73] Drolet, M., et al., Population-level impact and herd effects following the introduction of human papillomavirus vaccination programmes: updated systematic review and meta-analysis. Lancet, 2019. 394(10197): p. 497-509.

[74] Vesikari, T., et al., A Randomized, Double-Blind, Phase III Study of the Immunogenicity and Safety of a 9-Valent Human Papillomavirus L1 Virus-Like Particle Vaccine (V503) Versus Gardasil® in 9-15-Year-Old Girls. Pediatr Infect Dis J, 2015. 34(9): p. 992-8.

[75] Petäjä, T., et al., Immunogenicity and safety of human papillomavirus (HPV)-16/18 AS04-adjuvanted vaccine in healthy boys aged 10-18 years. J Adolesc Health, 2009. 44(1): p. 33-40.

[76] Reisinger, K.S., et al., Safety and persistent immunogenicity of a quadrivalent human papillomavirus types 6, 11, 16, 18 L1 virus-like particle vaccine in preadolescents and adolescents: a randomized controlled trial. Pediatr Infect Dis J, 2007. 26(3): p. 201-9.

[77] Lin, S.W., et al., HPV16 seropositivity and subsequent HPV16 infection risk in a naturally infected population: comparison of serological assays. PLoS One, 2013. 8(1): p. e53067.

[78] Olsson, S.E., et al., Induction of immune memory following administration of a prophylactic quadrivalent human papillomavirus (HPV) types 6/11/16/18 L1 virus-like particle (VLP) vaccine. Vaccine, 2007. 25(26): p. 4931-9.

[79] Human papillomavirus vaccines: WHO position paper, May 2017-Recommendations. Vaccine, 2017. 35(43): p. 5753-5755.

[80] Quadrivalent vaccine against human papillomavirus to prevent high-grade cervical lesions. N Engl J Med, 2007. 356(19): p. 1915-27.

[81] Walboomers, J.M., et al., Human papillomavirus is a necessary cause of invasive cervical cancer worldwide. J Pathol, 1999. 189(1): p. 12-9.

[82] Bonde, U., et al., Is HPV vaccination in pregnancy safe? Hum Vaccin Immunother, 2016. 12(8): p. 1960-1964.

[83] Harrison, R. and W. Huh, Occupational Exposure to Human Papillomavirus and Vaccination for Health Care Workers. Obstet Gynecol, 2020. 136(4): p. 663-665.

[84] Romanowski, B., et al., Sustained efficacy and immunogenicity of the human papillomavirus (HPV)-16/18 AS04-adjuvanted vaccine: analysis of a randomised placebo-controlled trial up

to 6.4 years. Lancet, 2009. 374(9706): p. 1975-85.

[85] Huh, W.K., et al., Final efficacy, immunogenicity, and safety analyses of a nine-valent human papillomavirus vaccine in women aged 16-26 years: a randomised, double-blind trial. Lancet, 2017. 390(10108): p. 2143-2159.

[86] Rowhani-Rahbar, A., et al., Longer term efficacy of a prophylactic monovalent human papillomavirus type 16 vaccine. Vaccine, 2009. 27(41): p. 5612-9.

[87] Slade, B.A., et al., Postlicensure safety surveillance for quadrivalent human papillomavirus recombinant vaccine. Jama, 2009. 302(7): p. 750-7.

[88] Kosalaraksa, P., et al., An open-label, randomized study of a 9-valent human papillomavirus vaccine given concomitantly with diphtheria, tetanus, pertussis and poliomyelitis vaccines to healthy adolescents 11-15 years of age. Pediatr Infect Dis J, 2015. 34(6): p. 627-34.

[89] Schilling, A., et al., Coadministration of a 9-Valent Human Papillomavirus Vaccine With Meningococcal and Tdap Vaccines. Pediatrics, 2015. 136(3): p. e563-72.

[90] Human papillomavirus vaccination coverage among adolescent girls, 2007-2012, and postlicensure vaccine safety monitoring, 2006-2013 - United States. MMWR Morb Mortal Wkly Rep, 2013. 62(29): p. 591-5.

[91] Syncope after vaccination--United States, January 2005-July 2007. MMWR Morb Mortal Wkly Rep, 2008. 57(17): p. 457-60.

Chapter 9

The Importance of the Extracellular Matrix in HPV-Associated Diseases

Joana Sampaio, Joana Ferreira, Ana Carolina Santos, Manuel Bicho and Maria Clara Bicho

Abstract

The extracellular matrix (ECM) is the non-cellular component of the tissues of our organism. It is the dynamic element that maintains a biochemical structure capable of supporting the organization and architecture of the tissue constituents. The diversity of ECM's constituents gives it the biochemical and biophysical properties necessary to regulate its behavior and differentiation. ECM has an important role in the biology of cancer cell development and progression. Human papillomavirus infection (HPV) is the principal etiological agent of the most common sexually transmitted diseases. It is a virus that can cause lesions precursors of epithelial squamous and glandular tumors. Type 16 (HPV16) is the leading cause of pre-malignant lesions and invasive cancers in these tissues. This work will focus on HPV infection to understand the role of ECM in the invasion, spread, and pathogenesis of the lesions caused by this virus. Cancer is no longer considered a pathology explained only by uncontrolled proliferation and apoptosis but also by the deregulation of the microenvironment.

The in-depth knowledge of ECM dynamics and its complexity is central and promising, specifically in developing new targeted therapies.

Keywords: Extracellular matrix, human papillomavirus, heparan sulfate proteoglycans, metalloproteinases, heparanase

1. Introduction

The extracellular matrix (ECM) can be defined as a three-dimensional, non-cellular macromolecular network made of collagen, proteoglycans, elastin, fibronectin, laminins, and other glycoproteins structural support for the organization of cellular constituents. It is known to be a physiologically active component of living tissue. The various parts of the matrix bind to each other and cell adhesion receptors, forming a complex network on which cells rely in all tissues and organs. Through transduction of extracellular signals originating from the ECM, cell surface receptors regulate diverse cellular functions such as survival, growth, migration, and differentiation and are vital for homeostasis maintenance [1, 2].

Each organ has a unique combination of elements in its constitution so that the specific function of the tissue itself can be fulfilled. This unique composition arises from biophysical and biochemical feedback between cellular components and the microenvironment, where they are inserted during the genesis of the tissue. The ECM continuously undergoes remodeling mediated by different decomposition enzymes, the proteinases being a highly dynamic structure. The balance between ECM degradation and secretion, orchestrated by ECM-modifying cells, is responsible for tensional homeostasis and organ-specific properties such as elasticity and compressibility [2–6].

In vitro, most animal cells have been shown to remain viable only when adherent to a substrate. Thus, the cell relies heavily on its sense of touch to survive by adhering and spatially interacting with the surrounding ECM- the concept of anoikis. The ability to attach and communicate with its environment is responsible for several growth factor receptors, and adhesion molecules arranged along the cell membrane, namely integrins. Indeed, cells have been shown to translate signals from the ECM to coordinate crucial morphological organization and signal events by regulating gene transcription. A cell converts external mechanical stimuli into a downstream intracellular chemical signal. This process is known as mechanotransduction. The sensitivity with which cells respond to biophysical and biochemical signals from the ECM demonstrates the importance of tissue homeostasis in maintaining healthy host cells.

Consequently, dysregulation of ECM remodeling has been shown to contribute significantly to cellular evolution through various fibrotic conditions, characterized by excessive ECM deposition and increased ECM stiffness. Due to increased interstitial pressure, irreversible loss of tissue homeostasis has been linked to an increased risk for various pathological conditions such as osteoarthritis, cardiovascular disease, and cancer [3, 4, 6–10].

2. ECM constitution

Various proteins that constitute the ECM result in different structures and properties. The main components of ECM include collagen, proteoglycans, laminin, and fibronectin. As each structure has a function, different subtypes and combinations of ECM molecules confer different functions essential to the correct functioning of the whole organism, **Figure 1** [11, 12].

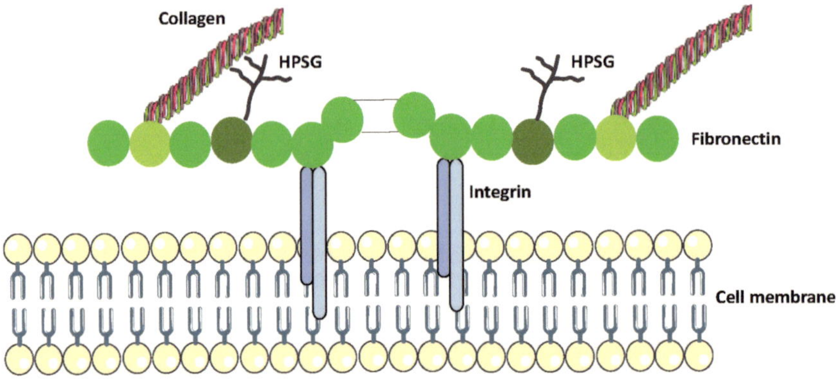

Figure 1.
ECM components and their organization. Organization of the different collagens, proteoglycans (HPSG), laminins, and fibronectin in the basement membrane and the extracellular matrix. In the basement membrane, laminin is attached to the cell, forming a fibrillar network. It is then linked to the type IV collagen network through nidogen and proteoglycans such as perlecan and agrinin. The different proteoglycans hold the fibrils together to form a collagen fiber. Fibronectin is bound to the cell by integrins and syndecans.

2.1 Collagen

Collagen is the basis of ECM architecture, is the most significant functional component, and the most abundant protein in human tissue. It can be classified into fibrillar (I-III, V, and XI) and non-fibrillar. Collagen fibers give ECM its tensile strength by limiting tissue distensibility. Collagens are trimeric molecules composed of three α-polypeptide chains that contain the sequence repeat (G-X-Y). This repeat allows the formation of a triple helix that gives the characteristic structure of this superfamily, **Figure 1**. Currently, there are 28 unique subtypes of collagen discovered. Each member of the collagen family has at least one triple helix domain. Most collagens bind to and interact with several ECM proteins forming supramolecular aggregates [3, 6, 8, 11].

Fibrillar collagens form fibrous structures often found in tendons, cartilage, skin, and cornea. Each collagen fiber is made up of several collagen subtypes in response to their tissue location.

Fundamentally we can define four classes of collagens:

1. Fibril-forming collagens (I, II, III, V, XI, XXVI, XXVII)

2. Fibril-associated collagens with interrupted helices (FACITs) (IX, XII, XIV, XVI, XIX, XX, XXI, XXII, XXIV)

3. Network-forming collagens (IV, VII, X)

4. Membrane anchored collagens (MACITs) (XIII, XVII, XXIII, XXV)

5. Short collagens (XXVI, XXVIII)

Types I, III, and V, predominantly produced by fibroblasts, are essential for the structure of the interstitial matrix. Their function as a pericellular "glue and structure" is necessary in tissue repair. Type IV is primarily located in the basement membrane and underlying epithelial or endothelial cells, ensuring their specialized polarization and function. Type IV collagen is the main constituent of basement membranes in tissues such as the lung, kidney, skin, intestine, and liver. It is mainly produced by endothelial and epithelial cells, and seen as intelligent collagen necessary for tissue repair processes that allow polarized cells (endothelial and epithelial) to survive and function, enable regular tissue function [6, 13].

2.2 Proteoglycans

Proteoglycans are the functional modifiers of ECM and provide additional properties. They are proteins characterized by being covalently linked to glycosaminoglycans (GAGs). These GAGs are long, negatively charged chains conferred by sulfate and carboxyl groups (heparan sulfate (HS), dermatan sulfate, and keratan sulfate (KS). The addition of sulfate and carboxyl groups to GAGs gives them this negative charge, enabling them to sequester water and cations (sodium and calcium) and have cellular lubrication and filling functions, **Figure 1** [6, 12, 14].

There are about three dozen extracellular matrix proteoglycans encoded in mammalian genomes, divided into several families. The two largest families include the LRR (leucine-rich repeat) proteoglycans and the hyalectans (such as versican). In addition to those mentioned, perhaps the most significant of all is perlecan (HSPG2), a multidomain protein that is part of all basement membranes. There are also two small families of transmembrane proteoglycans: glypicans and syndecans, both of which have heparan sulfate side chains, as does CD44 [12, 14].

Syndecans are encoded by four different genes and represent the most abundant transmembrane heparan sulfate proteoglycans (HSPGs). Their core protein comprises an extracellular domain, a single transmembrane domain, and a short cytoplasmic domain that interacts with the cell cytoskeleton. Glypicans are encoded by six different genes and are anchored to the cell membrane via glycosylphosphatidylinositol (GPI). The multiple organs of the human body contain different isoforms of HSPG with various polysaccharide compositions and sulfation patterns [12, 15].

The extracellular domain of syndecans is intrinsically disorganized, a feature that allows it to interact with a huge variety of molecules and perform a wide variety of biological functions. Some of these functions involve acting as co-receptors for tyrosine kinase receptors linked to growth factors. The HS chains of these proteoglycans share various ligands, such as matrix proteins, growth factors, cytokines, and chemokines, which are presented to high-affinity receptors present on the cell surface [3, 4, 6, 10].

In conclusion, proteoglycans are highly variable in their shape and structure to exert different functions in the ECM, i.e., and they are highly pleiotropic. This characteristic makes them essential in maintaining a healthy ECM, and without them, its entire structure would collapse.

2.3 Laminins

Laminins are trimeric glycoproteins formed by α, β, and γ chains often found in the basal lamina and mesenchymal compartments. The three chains form a coiled α-helical structure that builds the long arm, while the three short arms are each composed of one chain. At the end of the long arm are five laminated G-type (LG) domains of the α-chain that serve as binding points for the cell. Integrins, dystroglycan, lutheran glycoprotein, or sulfated glycolipids bind to these LG domains. At the end of each short arm are the N-terminal laminin (LN) domains that are important for laminin polymerization and the formation of the basement membrane [5, 6, 11].

Laminins have cell-specific functions such as adhesion, differentiation, migration, maintenance of phenotype, and resistance to apoptosis (anoikis). By binding to integrins, laminins can create a dynamic link between the cell and the ECM. The unique heterotrimeric laminins have the integrins as anchored partners allowing the induction of signaling pathways and the organization of the intracellular cytoskeleton. It has been observed that heparan sulfates directly mediate the interaction between laminins and collagen IV. Laminins play crucial roles in both basal membrane formation and interactions between cells and the ECM. While collagen, proteoglycans, and hyaluronic acid constitute the main structural component of the MEC, laminins are one of the molecules that bridge the cell-ECM interaction gap [6, 11, 12, 14].

2.4 Fibronectin

Fibronectin is a high molecular weight protein composed of two subunits linked together by two cysteine persulfide bonds. It is secreted in a soluble form by hepatocytes into the bloodstream or expressed in tissues by fibroblasts, forming a fibrillar network. The structure of fibronectin and its multiple post-translational modifications result in an immense variety of interactions with various ECM components (growth factors and GAGs) that mediate cell attachment and motility, ECM remodeling, host-pathogen interactions, among others. A single gene encodes this glycoprotein with 20 human isoforms resulting from alternative mRNA excisions (primary transcript). Similar to collagen, fibronectin forms a fibrillar network in the ECM. The structure of the fibronectin matrix is mediated by selective binding to α5β1 integrins. Compact, soluble fibronectin is secreted and unfolded through these integrins, revealing specific binding sites for other fibronectin molecules to form its fibrillar network. Binding to fibronectin induces integrin aggregation, which provides high local concentrations of fibronectin on the cell surface. This phenomenon promotes fibronectin–integrin interactions through the N assembly domains of each molecule [5, 6, 16].

Once fibronectin is attached to the cell surface by integrins, the actin cytoskeleton can drag molecules to the fibronectin to change its conformation. This will affect the C-terminal regions of fibronectin, revealing binding sites for fibronectin, heparan sulfates, heparin, collagen, and other ECM molecules. Through strong non-covalent protein–protein interactions, the fibronectin network matures and becomes insoluble, although other ECM proteins can mediate mature lateral interactions between fibrils. These interactions stabilize the relatively weaker binding sites [5, 6, 16].

In conclusion, fibronectin works as a skeleton upon which the bioavailability and activity of various growth factors are orchestrated. The interaction of fibronectin with growth factors (e.g., TGF-β, PDGF, HGF, VEGF, FGF) can impact cell migration, cell proliferation, survival signals, and angiogenesis as downstream outcomes of their activation through mechanical or enzymatic activation [5, 6, 14, 16].

3. Functions of the extra cellular matrix

The countless unique molecules that are part of the constitution of ECM give it various functions that simultaneously influence biochemical and biophysical processes in the cell. Although ECM was for many years considered an inert component that only provided structure to cells in tissue formation, its role in determining cellular functions and phenotypes has been clarified in the last two decades [2, 6, 14, 17].

The many proteolytic processes that modify ECM, by the action of proteolytic enzymes, play roles in ECM remodeling and are thought to release ECM-binding growth factors and expose cryptic activities in ECM, including the release of anti-angiogenic factors. Similarly, enzymes that degrade GAGs, such as heparanases and sulfatases, can also change the properties of proteoglycans in the ECM. Remodeling of the ECM by these various processes has important effects on development and associated pathologies [2, 14, 17].

Finally, ECM is known to transmit mechanical signals to cells and activate intracellular signaling mechanisms and the cytoskeleton machinery. The importance of ECM and its varied functions in the development and maintenance of cellular balance or homeostasis is indisputable [2, 14, 17].

3.1 Migration and proliferation

Cell migration is essential for tissue development, a fact demonstrated by neural crest cells, which migrate from the periphery of the neural tube to different parts of the embryo to form the heart, nerves, skin, and skull [2, 6].

The ECM influences the path and speed of migrating cells through its topography, composition, and physical properties. Cells migrate from regions with low ECM concentration to high ECM concentrations due to an adhesion gradient called haptotaxis. Proteases that degrade ECM also play a facilitating role in cell migration through a process involving matrix metalloproteinases (MMPs), their inhibitors, among other enzymes. It is essential to realize that constant remodeling of the ECM occurs during development [2, 4, 6].

3.2 Development

The topographic variation in the structure and elasticity of ECM provides cells with the ability to adapt and form complex morphological systems that are essential for different organs [2, 4, 6].

ECM modulates tissue growth to form complex structures that are necessary for these organs to function. In addition, it provides structural organization not only through its action as a physical barrier to cell growth and by activating intracellular signaling in a time- and context-dependent manner. ECM exerts this effect by modulating the distribution of growth factors, physical anisotropy, and anchoring [2, 4, 6, 11].

ECM also has an essential role in highlighting the influence on cell fate. This role is shown in mammary gland differentiation. Even with hormonal stimulation in vitro, mammary gland cells do not secrete milk proteins. However, after exposure of these cells to laminin-1, they begin to secrete these proteins. This phenomenon indicates to us that an appropriate ECM microenvironment is indispensable for the cell to be able to fulfill its functions [2, 4, 6].

To conclude, cells can sense the physical properties of the adjacent matrix and activate the appropriate intracellular mechanisms for their differentiation. Therefore, the physical properties of the ECM have cell differentiation capabilities.

3.3 Tissue homeostasis

ECM is a highly dynamic structure. Even after development, ECM is constantly being deposited, degraded, and modified to maintain tissue homeostasis. This is especially important for preserving cell phenotype and physiological processes such as wound healing, angiogenesis, and bone remodeling [2, 4, 6].

To maintain tissue homeostasis, cells in contact with the ECM perceive ECM properties through receptors and adhesion complexes. In turn, the cell regulates the expression of ECM components and enzymes based on the signals it receives. This leads to a feedback mechanism in which cell also influences ECM, resulting in a balance of deposition and degradation of ECM components [2, 3, 6].

The response of cells to other stimuli is ultimately influenced by the ECM components. The complexity and importance of the feedback mechanism between the ECM and the cell is essential to maintain tissue homeostasis [2, 3, 6].

The imbalance in ECM deposition and degradation leads to disease and is a hallmark of cancer and other conditions that course with fibrosis. Overall, the role of ECM in tissue homeostasis is to direct the appropriate cellular response and phenotype to maintain mechanical integrity and tissue function [6].

4. ECM disruption in cancer progression

Traditional views of cancer have been changing, and the significant role of ECM in the regulation of cell proliferation, migration, and apoptosis have been highlighted. At the microscopic level, the organization of ECM constituents forms a specific microenvironment that plays a critical role in tumor progression. ECM is constantly remodeling and actively influences cell adhesion and migration. Thus, small changes in the homeostasis of the microenvironment can result in significant effects on cancer cell proliferation. As the main component of ECM, collagen, dictates the main properties of the matrix, changes in its deposition or degradation can lead to loss of ECM homeostasis [2–4, 6, 11].

As cancer cells proliferate, the surrounding matrix changes a dynamic interaction between cells and the microenvironment. Changes such as increased fibronectin secretion, collagen type I, II and IV, indicate that tumor progression requires continuous interaction between the ECM and tumor cells. Increased deposition of matrix proteins promotes tumor progression as it interferes with cell–cell adhesion, cell polarity, and the amplification of growth factor signaling. High collagen deposition has been shown to result in tumor progression through increased integrin signaling [6].

The increased stiffness of the matrix activates integrins as well as cytoskeletal tension, promoting cell adhesion and motility [2–4, 6, 11]. It has been observed that local cell invasion of tumors is directed along collagen fibers aligned, suggesting that this linearization of the fibers facilitates invasion. These densely aligned collagen fibers are believed to act as cues for proliferating neoplastic cells to migrate outward from the tumor [2–4, 6, 11].

Tumor tissue hydration also has some impact on ECM dysregulation. Since it is strongly influenced by specific tissue GAGs due to their anionic structure and their ability to attract water, it is known that as hydration increases, the increase in intra-tumor hydrostatic pressure also increases, altering the biomechanical properties of the tissue that are known to be crucial for invasion [2–4, 6, 11].

Elevated levels of hyaluronic acid (carboxylated and free glycosaminoglycan) in ECM correlate with an increased likelihood of malignancy and poor prognosis. As a ubiquitous linear polysaccharide, hyaluronic acid (HA) is fundamental in determining the compressive properties of most biological tissues. Combining tensile strength due to collagen conformation and compressive strength due to hyaluronic acid creates the ideal biophysical properties for tissue homeostasis. Furthermore, hyaluronic acid is an induction signal for epithelial-mesenchymal transition (EM) and a migration substrate. It is also important in regulating vascular endothelial barrier permeability by stabilizing cell–cell junctions [2–4, 6, 11, 18].

Although increased levels of collagen directly promote ECM stiffness and mechanistically drive cell motility and proliferation, the exact role of hyaluronic acid in cancer metastasis remains unclear. However, its downregulation may serve as a key biomarker for invasion and metastization [2–4, 6, 11, 18].

5. Human papillomavirus (HPV)

5.1 The virus

The human papillomavirus (Human papillomavirus-HPV) is a small (55 nm) non-enveloped virus that belongs to the Papillomaviridae family. It can be classified according to its tropism (cutaneous, mucocutaneous, and mucosal). Since the availability of cellular factors expressed in different layers of the epithelium plays a role in viral gene expression and genome amplification, the viral cycle is strictly dependent on the epithelial differentiation program HPV infections are associated with some hyperproliferative pathologies of epithelia and mucosa, and most cervical cancer and warts cases. It has been described more than 200 types of HPV. Almost 40 types exhibit a particular tropism for the anogenital region's cellular floor epithelium and mucous membranes. HPV types in this subgroup are classified as being of high or low oncogenic risk, depending on the clinical lesions they cause.

The high-risk HPV types are associated with almost all cases of cervical cancer, and the low-risk HPV types are the cause of nearly all anogenital warts and low-grade lesions with a slight tendency for malignant progression. The most prevalent high-risk HPVs are HPV16 and HPV18, while the most common low-risk types are HPV6 and HPV11. Infections with specific high-risk HPV types are etiologically related to a significant proportion of vulvar, vaginal, anal, penile, and head and neck carcinomas [19–22].

5.2 Structure of HPV

HPV is a double-stranded circular DNA virus with 6.8–8.4 kb and can be divided into three functional regions:

- Early region (E-early), consisting of the early genes (E1-E8) that encode the replication proteins and regulate the different phases of the viral cycle.

- Late region (L-late) consisting of the L1 and L2 genes that encode the capsid proteins. L1 is called the major capsid protein and is responsible not only for the specific adhesion of the virus to the cell but also for the immune response produced by the host against this virus. L2, the minor capsid protein, appears to be important in the encapsidation of viral DNA [23].

- The long control region (LCR- long control region), consisting of regulatory genes, contains the origin of replication and the E6 and E7 genes that control transcription and regulate the expression of different HPV genes [19, 24].

The two oncogenes, E6 and E7, play a major role in carcinogenesis, contribute to immortalizing normal human keratinocytes in cell culture systems, and are essential to maintain the transformed phenotype in vivo. The main role of these proteins during the HPV cycle is to generate a permissive cellular microenvironment for viral replication. This includes the induction of DNA replication machinery, immune evasion, and the downregulation of apoptosis. To achieve this, the E6 and E7 proteins give rise to critical cellular regulatory pathways, including those dominated by p53 and pRb. The E6 protein (16–19 kDa) associates with p53 (tumor suppressor protein) and promotes its degradation. E7 (10–14 kDa) inactivates the function of another tumor suppressor protein, the retinoblastoma protein (pRB). Together, these two proteins promote the mechanisms involved in the genesis of tumors caused by these viruses, favoring cell transformation and immortalization [19, 24].

5.3 Viral replication

As already described, the life cycle of this virus is synchronized with cell differentiation and division.

Whether or not the viral life cycle is complete depends on the nature of the epithelial site where infection occurs and external factors such as hormones and cytokines. It is suggested that infection requires access to the viral particles (composed of viral DNA and the capsid proteins, L1 and L2) to the basal lamina and their interaction with HSPGs laminin [23]. Structural changes in the virion capsid facilitate transfer to a secondary receptor in the basal keratinocyte, necessary for virus internalization and subsequent transfer of the viral genome to the nucleus. Once internalized, virions undergo endosomal transport and pass into the nucleus, where the capsid disassembles and DNA release occurs. The L2-DNA protein complex ensures the correct nuclear entry of the viral genomes, while the L1 protein is retained in the endosome and ultimately subject to lysosomal degradation [20, 23, 24].

Infection is thought to require an epithelial wound or micro-wound to allow the virus access to the basal lamina. Indeed, active cell division, as occurs during wound healing, is required to enter the virus genome into the nucleus. It has been proposed that lesion formation requires the initial infection of a mitotically active cell [19, 20].

It is also known that in the basal cells of the epithelium, the expression of viral genes is repressed and expression of early (E) and late (L) genes only happens at the level of keratinocytes or the upper mucosal layers. Viral replication is associated with excessive cell proliferation of all epidermal layers except the basal layer. Since the basal cells of the stratified sidewalk epithelium are the only ones capable of dividing, they are the initial target of HPV infection [19, 20, 23].

Regardless of the nature of the infected basal cell, infection is followed by an initial phase of genome amplification and then the maintenance of the viral episode at a low copy number. The viral replication proteins E1 and E2 are considered essential for this initial amplification phase. The precise role of the HPV E6 and E7 proteins in infected basal cells is uncertain, particularly for low-risk HPV types that are not generally associated with neoplasia and whose viral DNA does not integrate into the chromosomes. They are thought to produce lesions following infection of a basal stem cell at the site of a wound. The role of the curative response in driving the initial proliferation of the infected cell may well be critical, with local microenvironment signaling influencing viral gene expression and/or protein functions. In the case of high-risk types that cause neoplasia, there is the integration of the viral genome into the chromosomal DNA, and the role of the viral E6 and E7 proteins in cell proliferation in the basal and parabasal cell layers is quite clear, especially at cervical sites where neoplasia can occur. It is clear that many functional differences exist between high- and low-risk E6 and E7 proteins and that these contribute, along with differences in promoter activity and gene expression patterns, to the different HPV-associated pathologies seen in vivo. Indeed, recent studies have suggested that a critical event in determining the neoplastic grade is the down-regulation of E6/E7 expression, even in the absence of genome integration, which is classified according to the extent to which basal-like cells extend into suprabasal epithelial layers. While such functional differences undoubtedly contribute to the respective abilities of high and low-risk HPV types to cause neoplasia and cancer, it is important to remember that a key function of the E6 and E7 proteins in most HPV types is not to promote basal cell proliferation but rather to stimulate cell cycle re-entry into the middle epithelial layers to allow genome amplification [19, 23, 24].

6. HPV-MEC interaction

As previously mentioned, the role of HSPGs in HPV infection is quite relevant [15, 25].

The HSPGs typically consist of a core protein and GAG chains. The core protein of syndecans is composed of an extracellular domain, a unique transmembrane domain, and a short cytoplasmic domain that interacts with the cytoskeleton. The glypicans are GPI-labeled HSPGs. The GAG chain comprises unbranched anionic polysaccharides composed of repeated disaccharide units formed by sulfated uronic acid and hexosamine residues [15–18].

As components of the ECM, HSPGs contribute to the organization of the basement membrane and mediate cell adhesion and motility. HSPGs bind to cytokines, chemokines, and growth factors on the cell surface, preventing their degradation, creating temporary storage sites or morphogen gradients important in development. Still, on the cell surface, they also serve as endocytosis receptors, and regulate the lysosomal degradation of extracellular molecules and provide nutrients to the cells. In addition, they are involved in the endocytosis of cell receptors. They mediate the transcellular transport of chemokines through endothelial cells. They also serve as co-receptors for a fibroblast growth factor (FGF) and its receptor. They mediate intracellular signaling or intracellular stress through the proteolytic shedding of syndecans and play an important role in developing and maintaining stem cell niches [15, 18].

The strategic localization of HSPGs in tissues is critical to their functional role. The localization of SDCs and GPCs at the plasma membrane regulates intracellular and cell-to-ECM signaling. The localization of HSPGs in the basement membrane regulates their barrier functions and coordinates cell–cell and cell-MEC interactions [15, 18].

Degradation of heparan sulfate chains by heparanase produces heparin-like fragments that activate FGF-2 mitogenicity. Therefore, the biological role of an HSPG depends on the properties of its core protein, the number of GAG chains attached, its location in cells and tissues, and the biosynthetic modifications that its GAG chains receive in situ. A wide range of biological functions is attributed to GAGs in cancer metastasis and other biological events due to their controlled, highly heterogeneous, and complex structure that allows for the regulation of tissue-specific functions [15, 18].

6.1 HSPGs as viral receptors

HSPGs are receptors hijacked by numerous viruses to bind to host cells. This typically occurs through electrostatic interactions between the negative charges of HSPGs and the basic amino acid portions of viral surface proteins. A consistent amount of data supports the natural dependence of HSV, DENV, and HPV on HSPGs for their binding to host cells [15, 26].

HSPGs, due to highly sulfated GAG chains, exhibit an overall negative charge that can interact electrostatically with the basic residues of viral surface glycoproteins or viral capsid proteins of non-enveloped viruses. Viruses exploit these weak interactions to increase their concentration on the cell surface and increase their chances of binding to a more specific entry receptor. HSPGs directly serve as entry receptors in rare cases, as described for herpes simplex virus (HSV)-1. Another study showed that HSPGs are crucial for SARS-CoV entry. Prophylactic treatment with bacterial heparinase I or heparin showed a reduction in SARS-CoV infectivity. Thus, either loss of HS or competitive inhibition confers some protection to cells against SARS-CoV. Given the structural similarities between SARS-CoV and the novel SARS-CoV-2, it would be interesting to study the effects of removing HS on SARS-CoV-2 infections. There are multiple ways to reduce viral contact with cell surface HS (HPSE, heparinase, heparin, soluble HS, and MMPs), investigating that this binding may give insight into SARS-CoV-2 entry and possible therapeutics [15, 26, 27].

All papillomaviruses are believed to rely on HSPGs for their initial binding. However, HPV-16 is the serotype whose pathogenesis is most studied due to its oncogenic potential and prevalence [15].

As already mentioned, the HPV infection cycle starts from the basal membrane of the vaginal mucosa, exploring abrasions or lesions in the epithelium (**Figure 2A** and **B**). The entry of HPV particles into host cells is a multistep process that begins with binding to HSPGs expressed on the cell surface of basal

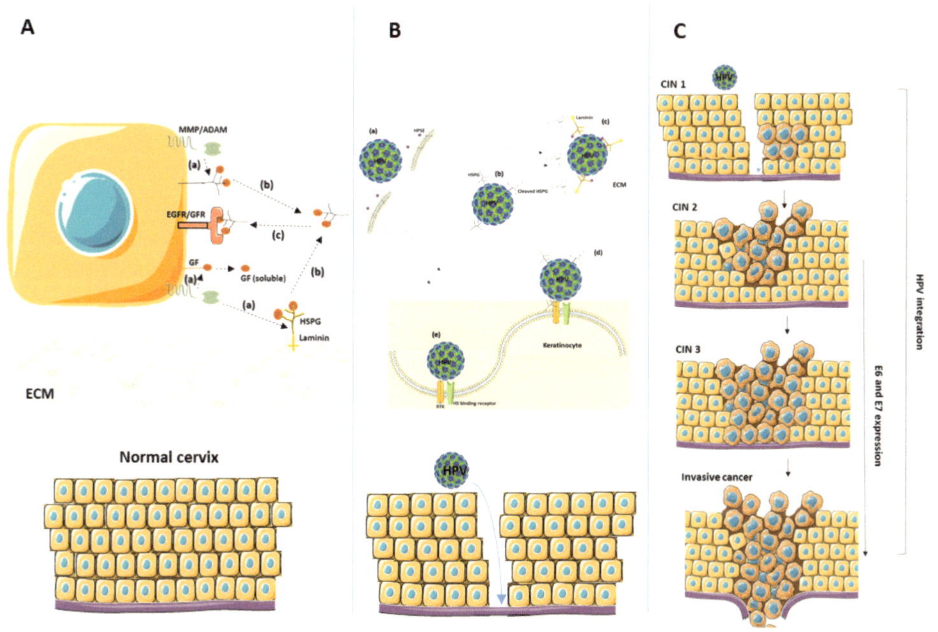

Figure 2.
Schema of the role of HSPGs in HPV16 infection. (A) Bottom is a normal cervix epithelia disrupted. Upper figure represents the details of wounded tissue healing mechanism, (a) MMP/ADAM cleaved GF (growth factor) bound to HSPG of cell membrane and also to the complex with laminin (b) shedd HSPG/GF complex, bounds to (c) adjacent cells GFR/EGFR as a co-receptor. (B) In bottom of figure HPV16 infected wound tissue release, as shown in upper figure, HPSE (heparanase) and HPV16 (a), HPV16 is coated with HSPGs and HS (heparansulfate) released respectively by MMPs/ADAM and HPSE, (b), HPV16 bounds to the complex HSPG-laminin in ECM, (c) adjacent keratinocytes through membrane EGFR-RTK and HS receptor bound as a complex (d) is endocytosed by the cell (e). (C) HPV16 integration by the infected keratinocytes during wound healing, after endocytosed in (B), progresses through CIN I, CIN II and CINIII to invasive cancer, after expression of E6 and E7 HPV oncogenic proteins.

keratinocytes or in the ECM. The interaction of the HPV16 L1 capsid protein with the HS chains of proteoglycans is well known but generally considered to have a passive role in infection. Binding to HSPGs induces conformational changes in the capsule and facilitates proteolytic cleavage of L1. This cleavage allows interactions between capsid and cyclophilin B, which results in further conformational changes that expose the N-terminus of L2. The exposed N-terminus contains a conserved consensus cleavage site for the extracellular proprotein furin convertase. This interaction is essential for successful HPV infection since cleavage of furin results in the exposure of a binding site on L1 postulated to be recognized by an unknown receptor. The described changes in virion conformation further facilitate the reduction in binding affinity to HSPGs, thus facilitating binding to the unknown receptor(s). These findings underscore the role of initial HSPG attachment to facilitate the critical step of L2 cleavage by furin and association with the putative second receptor for entry. Cleavage of furin has also been implicated in successful endosomal escape before transporting the viral L2/ADN complex into the nucleus, emphasizing the necessity of furin cleavage for successful HPV infection [15, 20].

Syndecan-1, the most abundant HSPG in keratinocytes, plays an important role in this initial binding due to its expression in epithelial cells and its overproduction during wound healing. It has been shown that syndecan-1 when released plays a major role in the infection of keratinocytes by HPV. Instead of separating it from its HS chains, HPV particles are released from the cell surface through the normal process of HSPGs, remaining bound to HS chains (heparan sulfate) and growth factors. They can bind to the epidermal growth factor receptor (EGFR). The specificity of growth factors is the bridge for the interaction of the virus with cellular receptors, for example, tyrosine kinase, whose signaling promotes infection **Figure 2A** and **B** [15, 28].

Considering the biology of HSPGs, it stands to reason that HPV particles bound to HSPGs would associate with ECM, and indeed, free syndecan forms bind tightly to ECM via their HS chains. Many studies have shown that HPV particles accumulate in the ECM, and LN-332, a component of the ECM, is a proposed attachment factor for HPV. There is already evidence of direct protein–protein interaction between HPV16 and LN-332 **Figure 2A** and **B** [15, 25, 28].

Thus, HS chain cleavage enzymes are known to increase the release and infectivity of HPV particles bound to ECM, indicating that many virus particles bind to ECM via these HS chains. Free syndecan-1 interacts with HPV16 and LN-332, demonstrating it to be an ECM-binding factor for HPV16, in addition to its role in binding HPVs to the plasma membrane. The interaction of snd-1 with LN-332 is expected based on reports demonstrating the concentration in the EMC of free snd-1 with its native HS chains and that LN-332 binds plasma membrane resident snd-1 with high affinity and specificity through HS chains. LN-332 has been identified as a binding factor between ECM and HPV. Since LN- 332 intrinsically lacks HS chains but contains HS-binding domains, it seems more likely that HS chains bridge the gap between HPV and LN-332, and this could account for the co-localization in the ECM of HPV and LN-332 **Figure 2A** and **B** [15, 25, 28].

Models have been developed for explaining the mechanism of HPV release from HSPGs:

1. It is suggested that conformational changes in the structure of the virus capsule are caused by the binding of HSPGs, which then allows cleavage of the HPV L2 protein, and subsequently triggers HPV release from binding factors that passively accumulate virus particles on their HS chains.

2. Based on the physiological processing of HSPGs molecules, HPV particles are released from the cell surface still in complex with HS and growth factors (GFs) and signal through GFRs to promote infection [28].

None of these models addressed ECM-bound virus release and infectivity. Still, a recent study suggested another model: high-speed processing of normal HSPGs from HPVs to gain infectious entry into keratinocytes. Inhibited viral release from ECM, cellular access, and infectiousness from ECM can be easily explained by this model. Proteases and heparanase play an essential role in HPV release from primary receptors [28].

This model, in which HPV usurps the processing of HSPGs and GFR/RTK signaling to promote infection, reflects the role of epithelial injury in mediating papillomavirus infections in vivo. Consequential breaks in epithelial damage result in an influx of HRs and cytokines involved in syndecan dissemination. Snd-1 expression is enormously increased in keratinocyte migration and proliferation, and free syndecans present in wound fluids regulate the activity of GFs and MMPs. Thus, HPVs appear to have evolved to control the epithelial wound to gain access to mitotically active basal cells and take advantage of the factors and architecture that favor infection. Many intracellular pathogens of the female genital tract (HIV, herpesviruses, chlamydia, Neisseria) interact with cellular HSPGs. Thus, it is tempting to infer that these pathogens also appropriate the biology of HSPGs during infection. In summary, there is new knowledge about the transmission of oncogenic HPVs, and high-speed pathogens usually function during infection of their hosts.

These findings may point to additional targets for preventing HPV infections and potentially those of similarly acting pathogens **Figure 2A** and **B** [28].

Upon contact with HSPGs, the HPV capsid undergoes conformational changes assisted by extracellular cyclophilin B and cleavage of the capsid protein L2 by furin. This leads to a loss of affinity for HSPGs and binding to different secondary receptors. Identification of the internalization receptor is ongoing, but α6 integrins, EGFR, and the tetraspanin family may be involved. The entry kinetics of HPV appears to be asynchronous and slower than for most other viruses, but the cause is not yet fully known. Some research suggests that it may be linked to the cell cycle phase or the involvement of multiple receptors. Subsequently, the virus is internalized through endocytosis, but there are conflicting reports on different HPV types and cells **Figure 2A** and **B** [15, 20].

The main goal in developing microbicides against HPV (or any viral infection) is to block the interaction between the virion proteins and the cell surface receptors used by the virus to gain entry into cells. As discussed earlier, the initial binding of HSPG is an important step for successful HPV internalization, as its inhibition has been shown to decrease HPV infection in vitro and in vivo. Since several different viruses use HS chains as the initial receptor/corrector to bind to the cell surface, it is considered a viable drug target, particularly about producing a microbicide with broad-spectrum protection against a range of HPVs (as well as other sexually transmitted viruses). Efforts in this direction will aid the development of antiviral drugs that are effective not only on many existing viruses but also on unpredictable emerging viruses [15, 20].

6.2 Pathogenesis and immunity

Once the basal layer of keratinocytes is reached, the virus can remain latent or take advantage of cell differentiation to replicate and initiate the disease. As for the host immune response, it is known that it can eliminate the infection or silence it (latent). The virus can persist with low infectivity, survive a weak immune response (persistence) and later induce pathology [19, 22, 24].

The mark of HPV infections is the effective evasion of innate immune recognition. The viral productive life cycle is exclusively intraepithelial, there is no viremia, no virus-induced cytolysis or cell death, and viral replication and release are not associated with inflammation. HPV globally decreases innate immune signaling pathways in infected keratinocytes, and pro-inflammatory cytokines are not released, activation signals to Langerhans cells, cell migration from and recruitment of stromal dendritic cells (DCs) and macrophages are absent or inadequate [19, 24].

Despite the high impact of HPV protein expression on cellular homeostasis, these viruses are incomplete carcinogens. Therefore, further changes in the cell and its microenvironment are required for tumor establishment and progression. This process includes dysregulation of the ECM. In some cases, changes in the levels and activity of defined ECM components have been experimentally associated with the expression of HPV-specific proteins, suggesting the direct involvement of the virus in the downregulation of these factors. Other studies, mainly those performed with clinical specimens, have identified changes in the levels of ECM molecules during the progression of HPV-related diseases [21, 29].

7. ECM alterations in HPV-associated diseases

The natural history of cervical cancer development begins with a precursor lesion called cervical intraepithelial neoplasia (CIN). CIN 1 CIN 2 lesions are classified as productive lesions, in which the viral cycle is complete. On the other hand, CIN 2 lesions and CIN 3 lesions are potential precursors of cervical cancer. The development of these lesions is mainly caused by persistent infection with oncogenic types of HPV. Intraepithelial lesions show low to moderate histological changes and may regress spontaneously within 1 to 2 years. In persistent high-risk HPV infections, high-grade precancerous lesions (CIN 2 and CIN 3) may develop within 3 to 5 years. Morphologically, CIN 3 (carcinoma in situ-CIS) represents a heterogeneous disease and can be considered a precancerous lesion of a more advanced cervical cancer **Figure 2C** [21, 30].

HPV infection has been associated with several changes in tissue organization and architecture, including downregulation of the expression and activity of MMPs. It has been shown that up-regulation of MMP-2 and MMP-9 expression and activity are associated with high-grade CIN, and their respective inhibitors have reduced expression levels in these lesions [4, 21]. On the analysis of MMP-11 and MMP-12 expression in high- and low-grade lesions, it was shown that both might be associated with the appearance of cancer precursor lesions and suggested that increased expression of these proteins may be considered an early event during the development of preneoplastic cervical lesions **Figure 2C** [21].

Alterations in other components of the ECM have also been explored in the context of cervical tissue transformation. Expression of the 67-kDa laminin receptor (LR67) was found to progressively increase with CIN grade. LR67 is associated with CIN 2 to 3 and can be considered a marker of cell proliferation in cervical tissue. These authors also demonstrated that combined analysis of LR67 and vascular endothelial growth factor-C (VEGF-C) could improve the clinical detection of high-grade CIN **Figure 2C** [21].

HPV infection has also been linked to a percentage of lesions in other epithelia of the anogenital tract, including the vulva, vagina, and anus. Vulvar, vaginal, and anal cancer precursor lesions are called vulvar intraepithelial neoplasia (VIN), vaginal intraepithelial neoplasia, and anal intraepithelial neoplasia (AIN), respectively. As with cervical precursor lesions, VIN and AIN also progress through degrees of epithelial transformation. The analysis of the expression of MMP-2, MMP-9, TIMP-1, and TIMP-2 by IHC in samples of VIN 1, 2, and 3 and invasive vulvar carcinoma suggested that overexpression of MMP-2, MMP-9, and TIMP-2 proteins may be related to the progression of VIN to invasive carcinoma **Figure 2C** [21].

8. ECM composition in HPV-associated cancers

The loss of regulation of ECM remodeling by unbalanced proteolysis plays a significant role in the loss of tissue homeostasis and pathological processes such as cancer. In cancer, this event may impact tissue tension and release chemotactic fragments of ECM components that influence the local microenvironment. It promotes cell migration and recruitment of stromal, endothelial, and immune cells to the tumor vicinity. The heterogeneous association of cancer cells and other elements observed in the tumor microenvironment, such as inflammatory infiltrate, endothelial cells, and tumor-associated fibroblasts, should also be explored to understand ECM remodeling changes fully [4, 21].

The most investigated proteases present in this process are the MMPs, as described previously. These MMPs play a central role in basement membrane breakdown and cell invasion and neoangiogenesis, and metastasis. Excess MMP activity generates topographical changes in the tumor microenvironment through modifications associated with proteolysis of the structural skeleton of the ECM. Indeed, linearization and thickening and/or degradation of specific collagen are common events observed in areas of epithelial tissue adjacent to tumor-associated blood vessels where cancer cells invade. The activity of MMPs also regulates cell migration and release of ECM fragments with biological functions, such as growth factors. The crucial role of specific MMPs in the process of carcinogenesis has set an objective task for researchers to explore the potential of MMPs as therapeutic targets. However, the use of broad-spectrum MMPIs offered no clinical advantages due to dose-limiting side effects [4, 21, 31].

Several authors have studied ECM alterations in both structural and remodeling molecules in invasive cervical cancer. More specifically, changes in the expression/ activity of galectins, collagens, proteoglycans, laminins, fibronectins, integrins, proteases, and regulators have been observed in cervical cancer samples derived cell lines [21].

The claudins (CLDNs) and occludins are families of proteins associated with tight junction establishment, epithelial cell polarity, and intercellular permeability. The expression levels of CLDN type 1, 2, 4, and 7 proteins are increased in HSIL lesions and invasive cervical tumors when compared with normal cervical tissues. On the other hand, occludin is expressed in the basal cell layer of normal cervical tissues. Its protein level is reduced in invasive cervical carcinomas compared with CIN samples. Thus, changes in cell adhesion and ECM structure are a common early feature in cervical cancer progression [21].

Expression of the high-affinity laminin-binding protein 67-kd (67LR) has also been shown to increase both CIN and cervical cancer samples compared to normal cervical tissues.

Versican, an ECM proteoglycan, was evaluated in cervical cancer samples by IHC (Immunohistochemistry) and situ hybridization (ISH). Expression of high levels of versican in tumor stromal myofibroblasts was associated with a lower frequency of CD8-positive T cells, more significant invasion and depth of tumor parametrial infiltration, and no change in cervical cancer survival. Interestingly, the beta-galactoside- galectin-1 binding protein was more expressed in stromal cells adjacent to cancer when compared to normal stroma associated with the cervical tissue. Furthermore, a higher expression level of galectin-1 was associated with increased local tumor recurrence and poor cancer-specific survival in patients with stage I-II cervical tumors after radiation treatment. However, it could not predict distant metastasis [21].

Laminin-1 and smooth muscle actin proteins (SMA) showed increased expression, mainly in the surrounding cervical tumor stroma compared to the normal cervical stroma. In addition, tumor cells especially expressed laminin integrin a6b4 receptors, and tumor-associated fibroblasts showed higher levels of laminin-a1 and laminin-b1 and lower levels of laminin-5, fibronectin, collagen III, TIMP-1, and the hyaluronic acid receptor CD44 when compared to normal fibroblasts. Finally, MMP-7 and MMP-9 expression has been shown to correlate with CD44 expression in skin cancer cells [21].

The data discussed above show that ECM composition and function alterations are common in HPV-associated lesions and cancers. Taken together, these changes highlight the complex molecular pathways that lead from initial infection to disease. For example, analysis of the impact of HPV on components of the MMP family has produced a spectrum of data that could be used for disease diagnosis and identification of targets for therapy. The data summarized here also show that, concerning the mechanisms by which HPV modulates MMP expression and activity, there is still much to learn. Finally, alterations in the ECM may impact the microenvironment of HPV-infected tissue, affecting the recruitment of inflammatory infiltrates, altering the fate of different cell populations present in the tumor, and ultimately determining disease progression and prognosis [4, 21].

More studies are needed to understand how HPV proteins affect the dynamic balance of the ECM in associated pathologies. This will help us to understand the disease genesis and define more appropriate clinical interventions. Importantly, the vast majority of the ECM changes described have also been observed in HPV-independent tumors. Therefore, understanding the virus-mediated molecular events that lead to ECM disruption may be useful for understanding the basic mechanisms of carcinogenesis and developing more general antitumor approaches [21, 32].

8.1 Heparanase and heparan sulfate/syndecan-1 axis

As mentioned earlier, syndecans are a family of four HSPGs that can be soluble or membrane-anchored. Syndecan 1 (SDC-1) is the one that has been most studied and is found mainly on the surface of epithelial cells. Loss of syndecan-1 and E-cadherin from the cell surface is known to be a critical step in the transition to epithelial neoplasia [18, 33].

The heparanase/SDC-1 axis is a key point regulating cell signaling when tumor cells are present and in their respective microenvironment. This heparanase/SDC-1 axis modulates cell proliferation as it regulates hepatocyte growth factor (HGF) and vascular endothelial growth factor (VEGF). HGF is a cytokine that increases the growth, motility, angiogenesis of tumor cells. Free syndecan-1 binds to secreted HGF and ultimately facilitates a paracrine and autocrine signaling cascade through the cellular receptor c-Met. It binds to syndecan-1 in the ECM, stimulating angiogenesis and tumor invasion via the Erk pathway secreted VEGF. To regulate gene expression, heparanase and syndecan-1 can also be transported to the nucleus to regulate gene expression. Overall, nuclear HS chains and syndecan-1 are considered anti-proliferative and decrease gene transcription. Specifically, highly sulfated HS chains are mostly inhibitory, contrasting with free syndecan-1 that promotes angiogenesis, proliferation, and cell invasion. Conversely, heparanase present in the nucleus increases gene expression and promotes growth. Thus, syndecan-1 expression is considered a prognostic tool in solid and hematologic malignancies. A high level of stromal expression of syndecan-1 is a negative prognostic factor, and low levels of epithelial expression are indicators of advanced disease and poor prognosis. Loss of syndecan-1 is believed to represent cancer cells with high malignant and metastatic potential [4, 17, 33].

9. Heparanase

Heparanase is an endo-β-D-glucuronidase that cleaves the side chains of HS. This results in the release of bioactive HS fragments from the ECM and in structural changes. Over the past two decades, much work has been dedicated to studying the role of heparanase in cancer biology. Various analysis methods have revealed that heparanase expression is increased in numerous cancers, including hematological malignancies, carcinomas, and sarcomas. In addition, elevated heparanase levels are associated with reduced postoperative survival, increased angiogenesis, and metastasis. All of these factors have triggered the development of heparanase inhibitors as novel anti-cancer agents [4, 17, 33].

Mammalian cells express a single functional heparanase enzyme, heparanase-1. Heparanase-2, a homolog of heparanase, has been cloned but cannot perform HS degrading activity. It can, however, regulate the activity of heparanase-1. The heparanase structure contains a TIM barrel fold, which incorporates the enzyme's active site and a distinct C-terminus domain with non-catalytic properties and is involved in the non-enzymatic signaling and secretion function of heparanase [17, 33].

The expression of heparanase is under tight regulation. In non-cancer cells, the heparanase promoter is constitutively inhibited, secondary to promoter methylation and p53 activity, which suppresses heparanase gene transcription by binding directly to its promoter. In addition, further regulation occurs during post-translational processing. Cathepsin L is required for post-translational activation of heparanase, and cathepsin L inhibitors prevent the formation of active heparanase. In non-pathological states, heparanase expression is restricted primarily to platelets, activated white blood cells, and the placenta with little or no expression in normal connective tissue or epithelium. In addition, it is most active under acidic conditions (pH 5–6), during inflammation, or within the tumor microenvironment [17, 33].

9.1 Role of heparanase in HPV viral pathogenesis

As already mentioned, increased expression of heparanase in numerous malignancies is associated with poor prognosis. And the direct role of this enzyme in neoplasms was confirmed when inhibition/silencing of heparanase in cancer cell lines resulted in a significant reduction in the invasive phenotype of the cells [4, 33].

The primary enzymatic activity of heparanase in the cleavage of the HS side chains of HSPGs and consequent release of growth factors and cytokines give rise to cell signaling pathways capable of inducing ECM remodeling. Heparanase can also release proangiogenic growth factors bound to heparan sulfates such as bFGF, HGF, PDGF, and VEGF, from the extracellular matrix to promote endothelial cell migration and proliferation indirectly. Tumors with high levels of heparanase have significantly higher microvascular density than tumors with low levels of this enzyme [4, 33].

Several heparanase capabilities have been demonstrated in the progression of cancers. These include increased cell proliferation via insulin, increased resistance to chemotherapy, expression of mesenchymal markers, increased autophagy, increased cell adhesion, and even a procoagulant function [26, 33].

Focusing on human papillomavirus infection, we remain to understand what role heparanase plays in HPV viral pathogenesis. Recent studies show that HPV16 particles bind to the ECM through HS chains. Reducing the activity of matrix metalloproteinases and heparanase drastically reduces the release of viruses from the ECM, which results in the loss of viral uptake and infection of human keratinocytes. On the other hand, exogenous heparanase promotes viral release and disease. This phenomenon may be necessary for explaining, especially at the wound site, the host healing response and RTK/GFR signaling that increases HS release, allowing an ideal environment for HPV to infect keratinocytes **Figure 2B** [3, 34].

Other research work has shown the significance of the HPV E6 gene in HPV-heparanase interaction in head and neck squamous cell carcinoma (HNSCC). The HPV E6 gene interacts with p53, decreasing its activity, leading to increased expression of heparanase since p53 is a potent inhibitor of transcription of this enzyme; expression of p21, a downstream component of the p53 pathway, correlates positively with heparanase expression on tissue section staining, confirming the heparanase-p53 signaling event. Polysaccharide segments of the HS chains serve as attachment sites for many growth factors, cytokines, chemokines, and various bioactive ligands. Cleavage of the HS chains by heparanase releases these bioactive factors increasing tumor invasion and malignancy in the case of HPV-induced HNSCC16 [3, 34].

10. The potential of future targeted therapies

Current statistics on the prevalence of HPV and cervical cancer alone underscore the need for alternative therapies to prevent and treat HPV infections. Existing HPV vaccines, while highly effective, do not offer protection against all high-risk HPV types, let alone low-risk HPV types. Furthermore, these vaccines are purely prophylactic and are not easily accessible to women in low- and middle-income countries (LMIC). For these reasons, alternative therapies that have broad-spectrum protection against HPV types, as well as other sexually transmitted infections, are worth exploring.

Since heparanase is an influential enzyme in tumor progression, it is the ideal therapeutic target. And since it is typically not expressed in healthy tissue, the side effects of its inhibition would be minimal. A series of heparanase inhibitors have been studied and produced, namely heparin, logically because it is a molecule close to HS. However, it is limited as an anti-cancer therapy because of its anticoagulant effects. Similarly, when LMWH (Low molecular weight heparins) was tried as an alternative for the same effect, but the results were controversial [4, 17, 33].

In addition to heparins, strategies have been developed to inhibit heparanase, such as HS mimetic molecules, modified heparins, etc. HS mimicking molecules have lower anticoagulant activity and greater selectivity for heparanase than heparin, allowing a wider therapeutic window. Some inhibitors already investigated are PI-88 (Mupaphosphat), PG545, SST0001 (Roneparstat), M402 (Necumparanib). In addition to HS mimetics, the non-steroidal anti-inflammatory aspirin, widely suggested to have a long-term anti-cancer effect, binds directly to the active site of HPSEs, inhibiting their enzymatic activity and preventing HPSE-dependent cancer cell migration, metastasis, and angiogenesis both in vitro and in vivo. As HPSE inhibition may seem attractive for cancer mitigation, it is important to note the critical role of the enzyme in the infiltration of activated NK cells in primary tumors and metastasis sites. Consequently, potential inhibitors must be highly selective and thoroughly investigated to limit adverse effects [4, 17, 33].

As we see, several heparanase inhibitors have entered clinical trials for various cancers, but none yet for viral diseases. Early results already suggest that using heparanase as a target may have rewarding benefits in controlling many viral infections, and thus the inhibitors listed above may have beneficial effects. Now, the promise that inhibiting this enzyme or the upstream effector, p65, could provide a novel therapeutic intervention to treat the disease. Overall, emerging knowledge about heparanase as an essential regulator of viral infections and associated morbidities could one day make a broad-spectrum antiviral drug a real possibility [34].

11. Conclusion

In this paper, we have discussed the extracellular matrix's very complex and important role in developing and progressing cancers and, more specifically, in human papillomavirus infection. Indeed, in recent years the ECM has been increasingly considered a crucial component in physiological processes such as cell proliferation, adhesion, and migration. The perspective of cancer and its progression has also changed. We no longer consider a disease caused only by dysregulated cell proliferation. Still, we give importance to the microenvironment and its changes and adaptations to cellular stress. In-depth knowledge of the ECM components, their complex interactions, and their constant and dynamic remodeling during all stages of tumor development brings some hope in developing promising targeted therapies to combat these pathologies. Likewise, knowledge of the components of viral particles and host cell entry factors and their specific interactions may allow the design of efficient antiviral strategies [15, 22].

Indeed, the role of HSPGs in HPV interaction with the ECM is undisputed and developed throughout the work. The enzyme heparanase, which we know has a significant impact on tumor progression and metastasis. Thus, as the influence of the tumor microenvironment on cancer progression becomes more evident, the focus on inhibiting enzymes that degrade HSPGs highlights an approach to maintain normal tissue architecture, inhibit tumor progression, and block metastasis. This review addresses the role of these enzymes, namely heparanase, in the context of the tumor microenvironment and their promise as a therapeutic target for cancer treatment, particularly cervical cancer [15, 17].

Acknowledgements

The Authors would like to acknowledge the Instituto de Investigação Científica Bento da Rocha Cabral for support.

Conflict of interest

The authors declare that they have no competing interests.

Acronyms and abbreviations

CD44	Cluster of differentiation 44
CIN	cervical intraepithelial neoplasia
CLDN	claudins
ECM	extracellular matrix
EGFR/RTK	epidermal growth factor receptor/ tyrosine kinase receptor
FGF	fibroblast growth factor
GF	growth factors
GFRs	growth factor receptors
GPI	glycosylphosphatidylinositol
HGF	hepatocyte growth factor
HNSCC	head and neck squamous cell carcinoma
HPSE	heparanase
HPV	human papillomaviruses
HS	heparan sulfate
HSIL	high-grade intraepithelial lesion
HSPGs	heparan sulfate proteoglycans
LN-332	laminin 332
LRR	leucine-rich repeat
LSIL	low-grade intraepithelial lesion
MMPIs	matrix metalloproteinases
PDGF	platelet-derived growth factor
SND-1	syndecan 1
TIMPs	an inhibitor of type 2 metalloproteinases
VEGF	vascular endothelial growth factor

Author details

Joana Sampaio[1], Joana Ferreira[1,3,5], Ana Carolina Santos[1,3,5], Manuel Bicho[1,3,5] and Maria Clara Bicho[1,2,3,4*]

1 Faculty of Medicine, University of Lisbon, Lisboa, Portugal

2 Institute of Preventive Medicine and Public Health and ISAMB – Environmmental Health Institute, Faculty of Medicine, University of Lisbon, Lisboa, Portugal

3 Genetics Laboratory and ISAMB – Environmmental Health Institute – Ecogenetics and Human Health Unit, Faculty of Medicine, University of Lisbon, Lisboa, Portugal

4 Dermatology Research Unit, Instituto de Medicina Molecular, University of Lisbon, Lisboa, Portugal

5 Instituto de Investigação Científica Bento da Rocha Cabral, Lisboa, Portugal

*Address all correspondence to: mcbicho@medicina.ulisboa.pt

References

[1] Reiland J, Sanderson RD, Waguespack M, Barker SA, Long R, Carson DD, et al. Heparanase degrades syndecan-1 and perlecan heparan sulfate: Functional implications for tumor cell invasion. J Biol Chem. 2004;279(9):8047-8055.

[2] Theocharis AD, Skandalis SS, Gialeli C, Karamanos NK. Extracellular matrix structure. Vol. 97, Advanced Drug Delivery Reviews. 2016. 4-27 p.

[3] Masola V, Bellin G, Gambaro G, Onisto M. Heparanase: A Multitasking Protein Involved in Extracellular Matrix (ECM) Remodeling and Intracellular Events. Cells. 2018;7(12):236.

[4] Piperigkou Z, Kyriakopoulou K, Koutsakis C, Mastronikolis S, Karamanos NK. Key Matrix Remodeling Enzymes: Functions and Targeting in Cancer. Cancers (Basel). 2021; 13(6):1441.

[5] Streuli CH. Integrins as architects of cell behavior. Mol Biol Cell. 2016; 27(19):2885-2888.

[6] Walker C, Mojares E, Del Río Hernández A. Role of extracellular matrix in development and cancer progression. Vol. 19, International Journal of Molecular Sciences. 2018.

[7] Buchheit CL, Rayavarapu RR, Schafer ZT. The regulation of cancer cell death and metabolism by extracellular matrix attachment. ScienceDirect. 2012;23(4):402-411.

[8] Ostapoff KT, Awasthi N, Cenik BK, Hinz S, Dredge K, Schwarz RE, et al. PG545, an angiogenesis and heparanase inhibitor, reduces primary tumor growth and metastasis in experimental pancreatic cancer. Mol Cancer Ther. 2013;12(7):1190-1201.

[9] Paoli P, Giannoni E, Chiarugi P. Anoikis molecular pathways and its role in cancer progression. Biochim Biophys Acta - Mol Cell Res [Internet]. 2013;1833(12):3481-3498. Available from: http://dx.doi.org/10.1016/j.bbamcr.2013.06.026

[10] Secchi MF, Masola V, Zaza G, Lupo A, Gambaro G, Onisto M. Recent data concerning heparanase: Focus on fibrosis, inflammation and cancer. Biomol Concepts. 2015;6(5-6):415-421.

[11] Iozzo R V., Gubbiotti MA. Extracellular matrix: The driving force of mammalian diseases. Matrix Biol [Internet]. 2018;71-72:1-9. Available from: https://doi.org/10.1016/j.matbio.2018.03.023

[12] Iozzo R V., Schaefer L. Proteoglycan form and function: A comprehensive nomenclature of proteoglycans. Matrix Biol [Internet]. 2015;42:11-55. Available from: http://dx.doi.org/10.1016/j.matbio.2015.02.003

[13] Karsdal MA, Nielsen SH, Leeming DJ, Langholm LL, Nielsen MJ, Manon-Jensen T, et al. The good and the bad collagens of fibrosis – Their role in signaling and organ function. Adv Drug Deliv Rev. 2017;121:43-56.

[14] Hynes RO, Naba A. Overview of the matrisome-An inventory of extracellular matrix constituents and functions. Cold Spring Harb Perspect Biol. 2012;4(1): 1-16.

[15] Cagno V, Tseligka ED, Jones ST, Tapparel C. Heparan sulfate proteoglycans and viral attachment: True receptors or adaptation bias? Viruses. 2019;11(7):1-24.

[16] Efthymiou G, Saint A, Ruff M, Rekad Z, Ciais D, Van Obberghen-Schilling E. Shaping Up the Tumor Microenvironment With Cellular Fibronectin. Front Oncol. 2020; 10(April):1-18.

[17] Hammond E, Khurana A, Shridhar V, Dredge K. The role of heparanase and sulfatases in the modification of heparan sulfate proteoglycans within the tumour microenvironment and opportunities for novel cancer therapeutics. Front Oncol. 2014;4 JUL(July):1-15.

[18] Elgundi Z, Papanicolaou M, Major G, Cox TR, Melrose J, Whitelock JM, et al. Cancer Metastasis: The Role of the Extracellular Matrix and the Heparan Sulfate Proteoglycan Perlecan. Front Oncol. 2020;9(January).

[19] Bicho MC. Microbiologia Médica - Cap 44. Virologia Médica (Editado por Helena Barroso, António Meliço-Silvestre, Victor Duque e Nuno Taveira). Lidel Edições Técnicas , Lisboa - 2014. ISBN:978-972-757-576-3

[20] Carse S, Bergant M, Schäfer G. Advances in targeting hpv infection as potential alternative prophylactic means. Int J Mol Sci. 2021;22(4):1-28.

[21] Herbster S, Paladino A, de Freitas S, Boccardo E. Alterations in the expression and activity of extracellular matrix components in HPV-associated infections and diseases. Clinics. 2018;73:1-7.

[22] Leto M das GP, Santos Júnior GF Dos, Porro AM, Tomimori J. Human papillomavirus infection: etiopathogenesis, molecular biology and clinical manifestations. An Bras Dermatol [Internet]. 2011;86(2):306-17. Available from: http://www.ncbi.nlm.nih.gov/pubmed/21603814

[23] R.Keiffer LGMGMB-HMSSDT. Human Papillomavirus Major Capsid Protein L1 Remains Associated with the Incoming Viral Genome throughout the Entry Process. J Virol. 2017;91(16):1-17.

[24] Doorbar J, Quint W, Banks L, Bravo IG, Stoler M, Broker TR, et al. The biology and life-cycle of human papillomaviruses. Vaccine [Internet]. 2012;30(SUPPL.5):F55–F70. Available from: http://dx.doi.org/10.1016/j.vaccine.2012.06.083

[25] Raff AB, Woodham AW, Raff LM, Skeate JG, Yan L, Da Silva DM, et al. The Evolving Field of Human Papillomavirus Receptor Research: a Review of Binding and Entry. J Virol. 2013;87(11):6062-6072.

[26] Koganti R, Suryawanshi R, Shukla D. Heparanase, cell signaling, and viral infections. Cell Mol Life Sci [Internet]. 2020;77(24):5059-77. Available from: https://doi.org/10.1007/s00018-020-03559-y

[27] Clausen TM, Sandoval DR, Spliid CB, Pihl J, Perrett HR, Painter CD, et al. SARS-CoV-2 Infection Depends on Cellular Heparan Sulfate and ACE2. Cell. 2020;183(4):1043-1057.e15.

[28] Surviladze Z, Sterkand RT, Ozbun MA. Interaction of human papillomavirus type 16 particles with heparan sulfate and syndecan-1 molecules in the keratinocyte extracellular matrix plays an active role in infection. J Gen Virol. 2015;96(8):2232-2241.

[29] Cogliano V, Baan R, Straif K, Grosse Y, Secretan B, Ghissassi F El. 4. Molecular Mechanisms of HPV-induced Carcinogenesis. IARC Monogr Vol 90. 2007;90:432-65.

[30] IARC WORKING GROUP. Human Papillomavirus (HPV) Infection [Internet]. Vol. VOLUME 90, IARC MONOGRAPHS. International Agency for Research on Cancer; 2010. 11-12 p. Available from: http://www.cdc.gov/std/treatment/2010/hpv.htm

[31] Branca M, Ciotti M, Giorgi C, Santini D, Di Bonito L, Costa S, et al. Matrix metalloproteinase-2 (MMP-2) and its tissue inhibitor (TIMP-2) are

prognostic factors in cervical cancer, related to invasive disease but not to high-risk human papillomavirus (HPV) or virus persistence after treatment of CIN. Anticancer Res. 2006;26(2 B): 1543-56.

[32] Oxford JT, Reeck JC, Hardy MJ. Extracellular matrix in development and disease. Int J Mol Sci. 2019;20(1).

[33] Heyman B, Yang Y. Mechanisms of Heparanase Inhibitors in Cancer Therapy. Physiol Behav. 2019;176(3):139-48.https:// doi. org/10.1016/j.exphem.2016.08.006

[34] Thakkar N, Yadavalli T, Jaishankar D, Shukla D. Emerging roles of heparanase in viral pathogenesis. Pathogens. 2017;6(3):1-12.